MOVEMENT
IS
MEDICINE
ANTHOLOGY

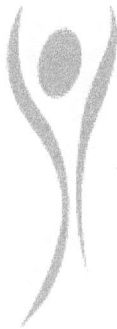

Published by RadiKal Publications, a division of

DIAMONDS WORLD INC

PO Box 5012

Wilmington De 19808

WWW.DIAMONDS-WORLD.ORG

ISBN: 978-0-9835917-4-0

Copyright © 2012

MOVEMENT IS MEDICINE

ANTHOLOGY

Editing: RadiKal Publications

Cover Graphics: New Media Dezigns

Printed in the United States: First Printing

MOVEMENT
IS
MEDICINE
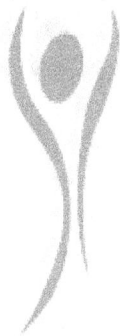
ANTHOLOGY

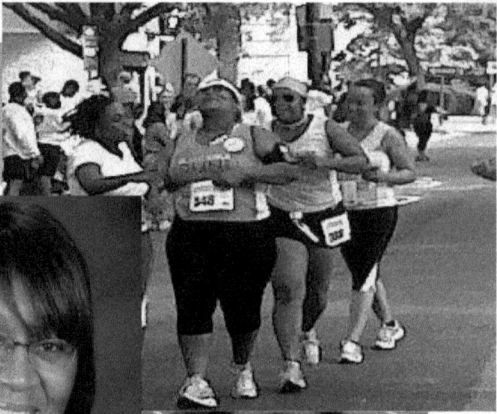

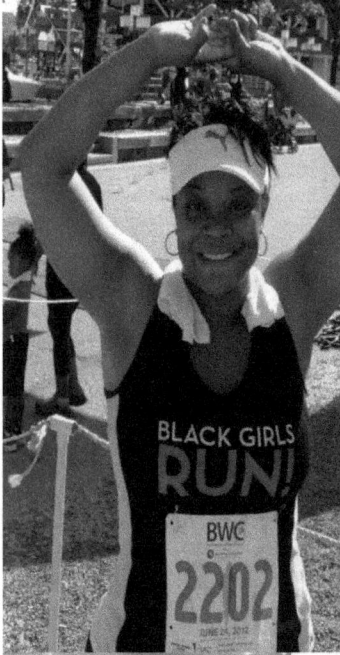

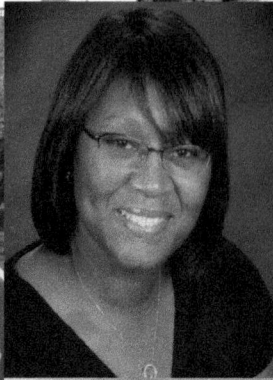

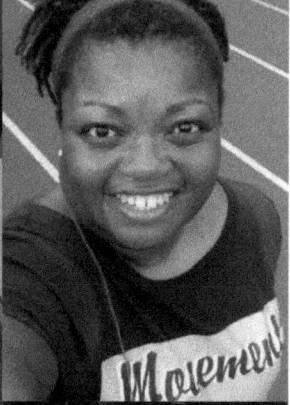

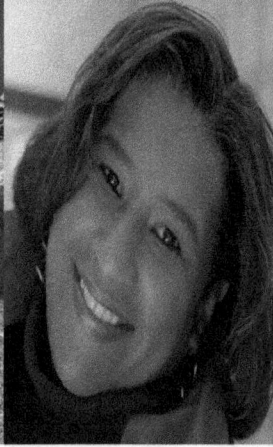

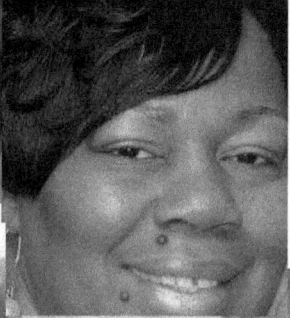

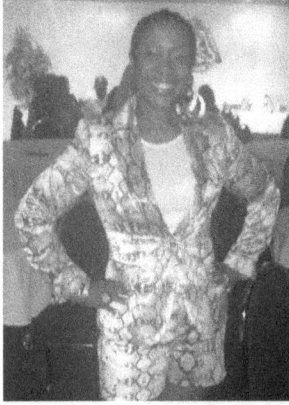

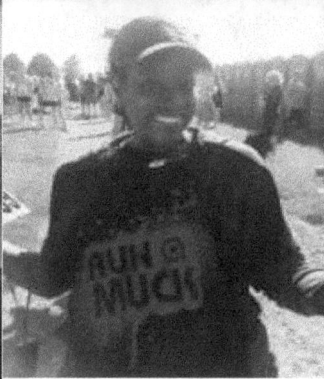

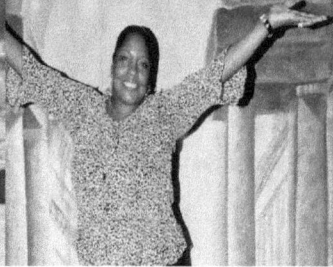

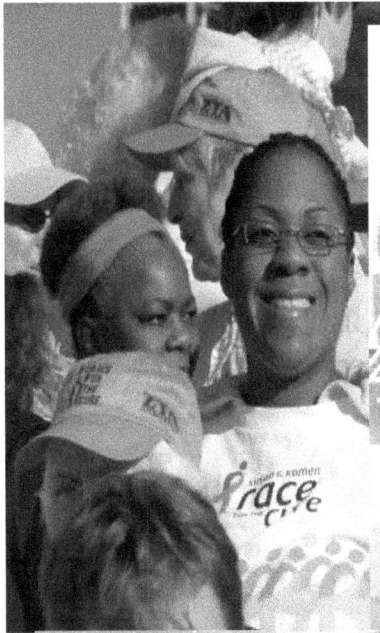

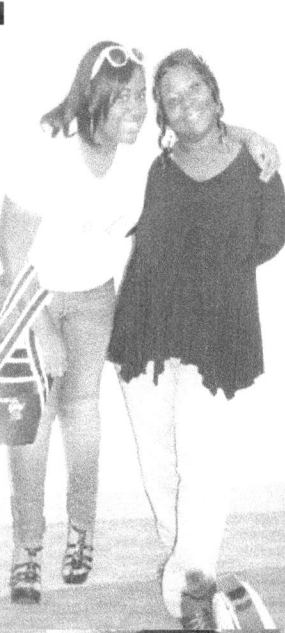

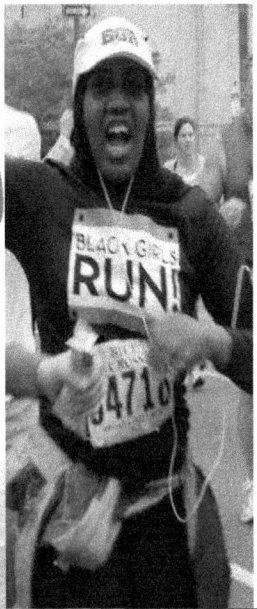

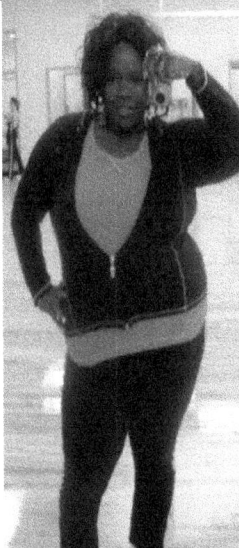

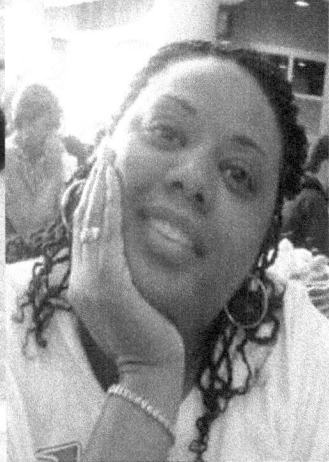

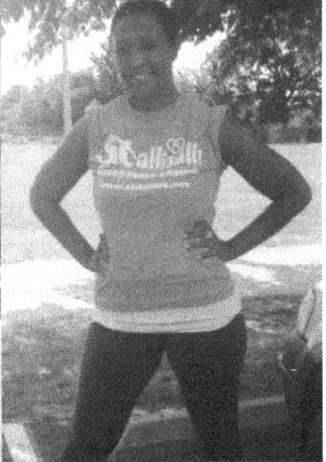

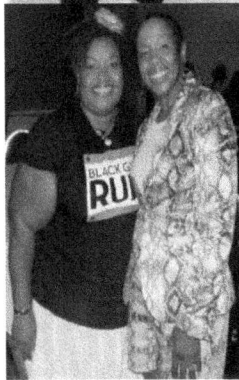

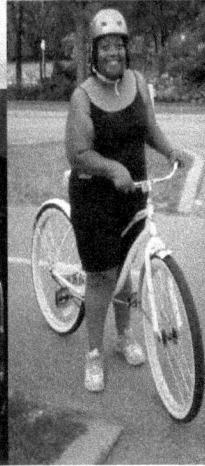

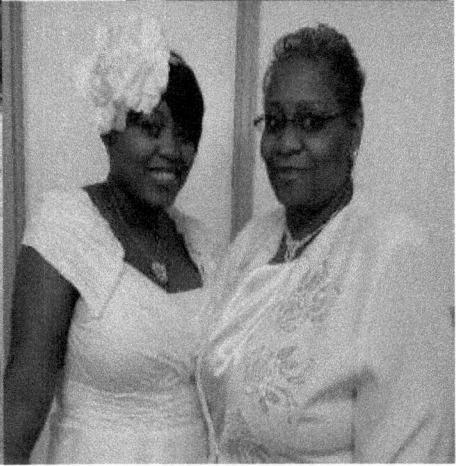

ACKNOWLEDGEMENTS

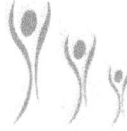

This book would not be possible had it not been for several wonderful people that I have met along my journey and we would like to pause and say thank you at this time.

First, we want to thank God for the wonderful work that He has done in our lives. He is the Chief Architect of it all. All creative concepts and rights come from Him and Him alone. We give Him all the glory honor and praise for everything. He is the giver of every good and perfect gift. To get the gift of your life and health back is awesome, and we as the writers of *MOVEMENT IS MEDICINE ANTHOLOGY* are grateful.

To David Rosario who prophetically spoke the words, "Movement IS Medicine" into my life one morning, I thank you. Those words changed and challenged my life. It has become the mantra for many for who are now getting up and moving. Words can never express my feelings of gratitude. THANK YOU for imparting your God-given words to impact and change the lives of people. God only gives gifts to those whom He can trust and He has found that He can indeed trust you! Be blessed my Omega Brother!

To all of the writers who contributed to this *MOVEMENT IS MEDICINE ANTHOLOGY,* thank you, thank you, and thank you again. You began to share your hearts and your stories and you made this project come alive. Many of you were already sharing your stories with us long before the concept of the book was conceived. It was as if God used you to say, "Look, let me help this project get started." In many ways you did. We are honored that you trusted us enough to share your hearts, your words and your stories in this project. It was a wonderful selfless act of wanting to extend a hand up to the next one that is coming behind you. They needed to know that they too can overcome any obstacle and reclaim their health; mentally, emotionally, and spiritually. They now know that they can bounce back and come out victorious! We celebrate you today for the gifts that you are to the world and for sharing your gift with the world.

To our publisher, Shirelle Diamond Hogans of Radikal Publications, we thank you! You did this in three days, the same amount of days that Jesus was crucified, buried and risen from the dead. That is an amazing feat and you should be proud of yourself. You were born to do this and we are so grateful for all the blood sweat and tears you put into this project for us. You worked tirelessly for hours and poured your love and care as if this was your own baby. For that, we are eternally grateful. Diva, you rock and we celebrate you for that gift that you are to the world. Continue to press forward and do great things!

FOREWORD

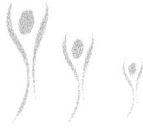

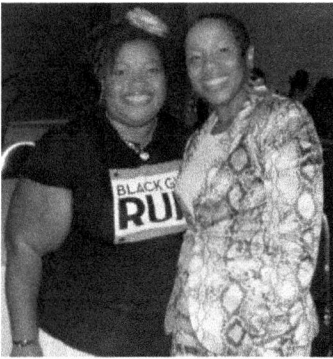

The two women you see in this picture are the kindred spirits that God Himself joined together in His divine wisdom because He had a plan. He had a destiny and purpose for their lives.

MOVEMENT IS MEDICINE ANTHOLOGY was birthed from various places. One of them was a conversation that Deneen Young and Ramona M. Gaines had one day that lead to many more. We both understood that if you truly want to loose the weight, it begins long before you lace up your first sneaker or your first day on the treadmill. It begins in your mind, because to truly get the medicine you really need, you must acknowledge that your lifestyle needs a total makeover.

We need to start by hitting the reset button. What does that mean? It means you have to be open to the renewing of your mind. Renewing your mind allows God to come in and deal with the issues of why you eat. Eating is also a form of self-medicating. Therefore, with that understanding, we must begin to delve deeper into our own personal issues if we want to get the results we so desperately say we want.

For Deneen and I, our journey began in the offices of therapist and psychologist. We understood that we needed to excavate the pain of the past to have the future we wanted. Not just for ourselves, but for our families as well.

We used the Word of God as a daily tool to strengthen and encourage us. Our consistency cancelled the negative thoughts of what people said we were and even what we believed about ourselves.

We learned about food; what it means to eat clean (no white flour such as white bread, white rice, increase fresh fruit & vegetable intake and grains) portion control, the nutritional value and how to use it as fuel for our bodies so that we could maximize our potential and live our best life. We were open to the instruction of those around us who shared their wisdom about strength training, muscle development and what it means to learn and listen to your body. We gained understanding on how the discipline of this new way of life would eventually spill over into other areas of our lives. It made us acknowledge and take ownership of other areas we needed to get in order. For example: finances, family time and time for God.

The lesson we learned in essence was BALANCE. We must have balance in our lives. No, we are not going to get it right all the time. However, as Paul said, "We press towards the mark for the prize." In Deneen's words, "We keep pressing and pushing everyday because Movement IS Medicine, on so many levels....."

We invite you to connect with *MOVEMENT IS MEDICINE*:

movementismedicine23@gmail.com
http://www.facebook.com/MovementIsMedicine

GET UP
AND *MOVE*
SOMETHING

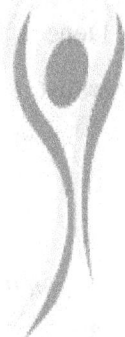

Introduction

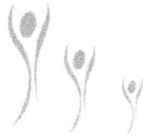

The "Movement Is Medicine" train is moving. We are leaving no one behind. What is the medicine? The medicine is moving; moving out of broken heartache and headaches, broken dreams, promises and people. Moving out of broken mental, emotional, physical, and spiritual places. Moving out of broken marriages, broken families, and broken people and not to mention, broken finances. Just plain broke. Why stay there? Why stay stuck? What are we moving to? We are moving to wholeness in every sense of the word; mind, body soul and spirit. We are calling back all of our parts that have been broken and splintered into perfect alignment and harmony unto ourselves. We are just like the lepers who were healed as they went, because the medicine was in the moving. It took faith to move, even when they could not immediately see it but they had to conceive it and then walk in belief. Today, ask God to cleanse your womb so that you may be able to carry this baby to full term. When you birth this one out, it will be full of purpose and promise. Moreover, the 'Pit' with all of its pain will no longer matter. All you will see is the beauty of the baby, the promise and manifested seed. The things that God said would happen.

TABLE OF CONTENTS

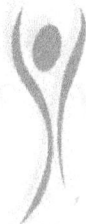

GET UP
AND *MOVE*
SOMETHING

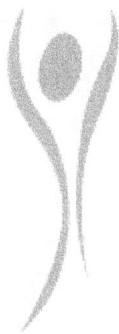

GET IN THE ZONE

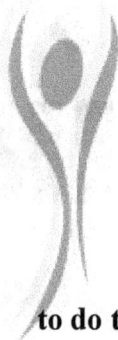

I fell in love with me!

MY bravery,

MY persistence,

MY confidence and

MY ability

to do the unthinkable and be ok with it.

JOYCE NICHOLE ROBINSON

GET IN THE ZONE

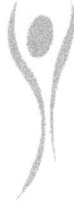

"I have chosen to be happy because it is good for my health"

    --Voltaire

Just when you think life if great, it isn't. Just when you think your problems couldn't get worse, they do. It's not always about what or who knocks you down, it's about YOU and how you get back up!

Over the past six months, I've learned so much. I've grown as a woman, a mother and a child of God. There is nothing on this Earth that could've prepared me for what happened. I am so blessed and thankful that my God was there all the time. He is the one who steadied me for the race that was to come. Daily, He puts me back on the right path when I veer off course.

Life as I knew it came to a screeching halt in early February 2012. After a little over eight years of marriage and being together a total of fourteen years, my husband decided that we should part. It was over! While I'd never use this opportunity to bash my husband or put our personal lives on display, I will say that our sudden break-up awakened something in me that had been buried since high school, my resilience.

I COULD NOT EAT!

I could not sleep.

I could not function.

My world was imploding and all I could do was pray that God would turn things around and spare me from the pain and anxiety that had taken over my world. For nearly a month, I could stomach nothing more than yogurt and weight loss shakes. I ate a few things here and there; sometimes I could hold it down and sometimes I couldn't. I was in a daze. To make things more challenging, I had started an entirely new career exactly a week before the "break up". It seemed as though I barely had enough mental energy to get to and from work. There was no way that eating was a priority.

Since I didn't really know anyone at my new job, no one noticed that I was rapidly losing weight nor did they notice that I wasn't eating. In order to socialize with colleagues, I'd go to the cafeteria to buy lunch but I never ate it. I'd take it home most days and attempt to eat it, but for the most part the food always ended up in the trash, barely touched.

In mid-March, after about six weeks, the fog began to lift. I was ready to accept that my marriage was over. While I was moving on from being a wife, I was still a mother. One day I lay in bed and I heard God say to me, "Get up, be a victorious mom, not a victim. Show those boys that you are strong!" I went into the bathroom and stared into the mirror. I saw a much thinner face, swollen cried-out eyes, and dry pale skin. I looked over my body and saw nothing short of a messy shell.

I got dressed for work and looked into a larger mirror. For the very first time, I saw a new ME! I saw a much thinner version of who I had become. My clothes were so big that even my belt couldn't hold my pants up! For the first time in a long time, I didn't cry. I smiled. I even laughed a bit. I had been trying for the last year to take off the weight that I'd gained since the birth of my youngest son. Little did I know the **"BREAK UP DIET"** would do the trick!

You see, years ago, after the birth of my first son, I looked at a holiday photo and what I saw repulsed me. I was fat! I was squeezed into clothing and I was uncomfortable. I decided to lose weight and change my life. I completely changed the way I ate, but I never exercised! I didn't think it mattered as long as the end result was major weight loss. I ended up losing so much weight that I had to consciously regain weight. Friends and co-workers were even calling me "Tyra Banks" and "super model". It felt awesome!

From that day in March forward, I decided to keep the weight loss going, but in a healthy way. I just picked up and started eating again. I went back to my healthy eating lifestyle and I decided to use my unwelcomed kick start as a way to get my "super model" back. However, guess what? The thought of exercise still repulsed me.

GET IN THE ZONE

As the weeks turned into months, I continued to be pleased with my healthy eating and weight loss. I gave myself a head to toe make-over and firmly committed to living MY life for me. One day, at the end of June, I received a Facebook message from a woman that I didn't know. The content of the message was about something foreign to me, RUNNING! I always delete messages from people I don't know, but I decided to read it. I think it was God. No wait, I KNOW it was God who intervened and made me read it. It was an invite to a new Black Girls Run (BGR) "meet-up" in my area.

I'd heard of BGR but obviously BGR hadn't heard that I don't (or at least didn't) do 'girlsweat!' I sat at my desk and stared out of the window and flashed back to all of the obstacles I had recently overcome. A soft voice floated through my head and said, "You're going to do this!" I looked around for the candid cameras. I laughed when there were none and said in a quiet voice, "Ok Lord. After all I've been through in my life and especially these last few months, I can do anything, huh?" With that notion, the desire to run was born.

MOVEMENT IS MEDICINE

I knew I was on to something when I felt that same desire that I had years earlier when I embarked on my first weight loss journey. I officially registered on the Black Girls Run website. I requested to be added to the private Facebook group and I went shopping for cute running outfits, of course! On July 3, 2012 I attended my very first meet up. I was immediately embraced into this group of strangers. These women didn't know me yet they encouraged me and lifted me up emotionally more than anything had in months!

I fell in love with me!
MY bravery,
MY persistence,
MY confidence and
MY ability
to do the unthinkable and be ok with it.

I know millions of women run every day. It's certainly not an Earth shattering concept, but for me it was. For the first time ever I didn't care about my hair, 'girlsweat', or what others thought of me. Of course I started out slow. I walked, I wogged (combination of walking and jogging), I jogged and I even ran a bit, but I DID IT! I just let go. In that moment, I knew that I needed to let go of all kinds of baggage.

I was totally free to be me.

I committed to hitting the track at least 2-3 times a week. It may not have been a lot but it was major to me. Not only did I begin to run, I began to exercise period! Every time I would hit the track, I'd enter what some folks call 'the zone'. I could think, rationalize, pray, cry and leave it all out there on the track. One day, I looked up and the day had turned to night. My pedometer indicated that I had gone five miles, and boy was I sore! While I had mostly walked those five miles I felt so much better mentally. I had so much on my mind and in my heart that I was beginning to feel suffocated.

I limped off the track that night with clarity.

I know that my journey isn't all that special. People's lives change every day. Marriages end all the time, I get that. However, for as strong as I had always been, I was broken and at times emotionally paralyzed. God told me to MOVE in more ways than one. I was commanded to MOVE from the place that I was in. I was not to stay as my flesh would have wanted. If I had been allowed to stay surely it would have been easier in a lot of ways. If I had never picked up a sneaker or shed a pound, it would have been easier. My body wouldn't be tired and I'd be able to hide my true emotions behind excessive eating.

If I had not MOVED EMOTIONALLY, SPIRITUALLY and PHYSICALLY, I would not be on the way to true and lasting healing. I'd be stuck! My journey and journeys like mine prove that Movement IS Medicine! It is medicine for the heart, the mind, the spirit and the physical temples that God has blessed us with.

"I can do all things through Christ who strengthens me."
Philippians 4:13

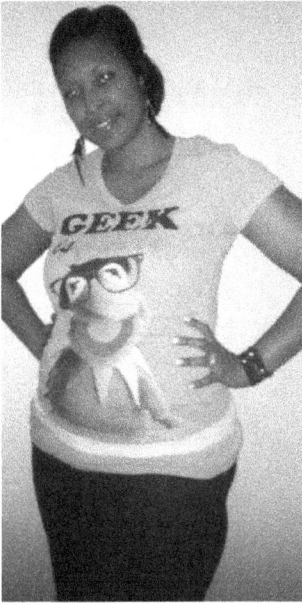

Joyce Nichole Robinson is a 37 year old mother of two sons, Bryson and Blaize. Creative writing has long since been a passion that Joyce loves to get lost in. Recently, with the burst of social networking, Joyce has fallen in love with blogging about topics such as health and wellness, motherhood, mentoring and relationships.

For nearly 20 years, Joyce has worked in the Human Service field in one capacity or another. From helping at-risk youth gain access to and learn to value education; to mentoring young ladies, reaching back and helping others has always been a priority.

Recently, personal trials have taught Joyce valuable lessons that she may not have otherwise cared to learn. Taking charge of her physical, emotional and spiritual well-being has given Joyce freedoms which she never imagined possible. Through her belief in God she has gained strength and knowledge to overcome tests and turn them into testimonies.

Movement—spiritual, emotional AND physical is a MUST for the soul. Movement IS Medicine!

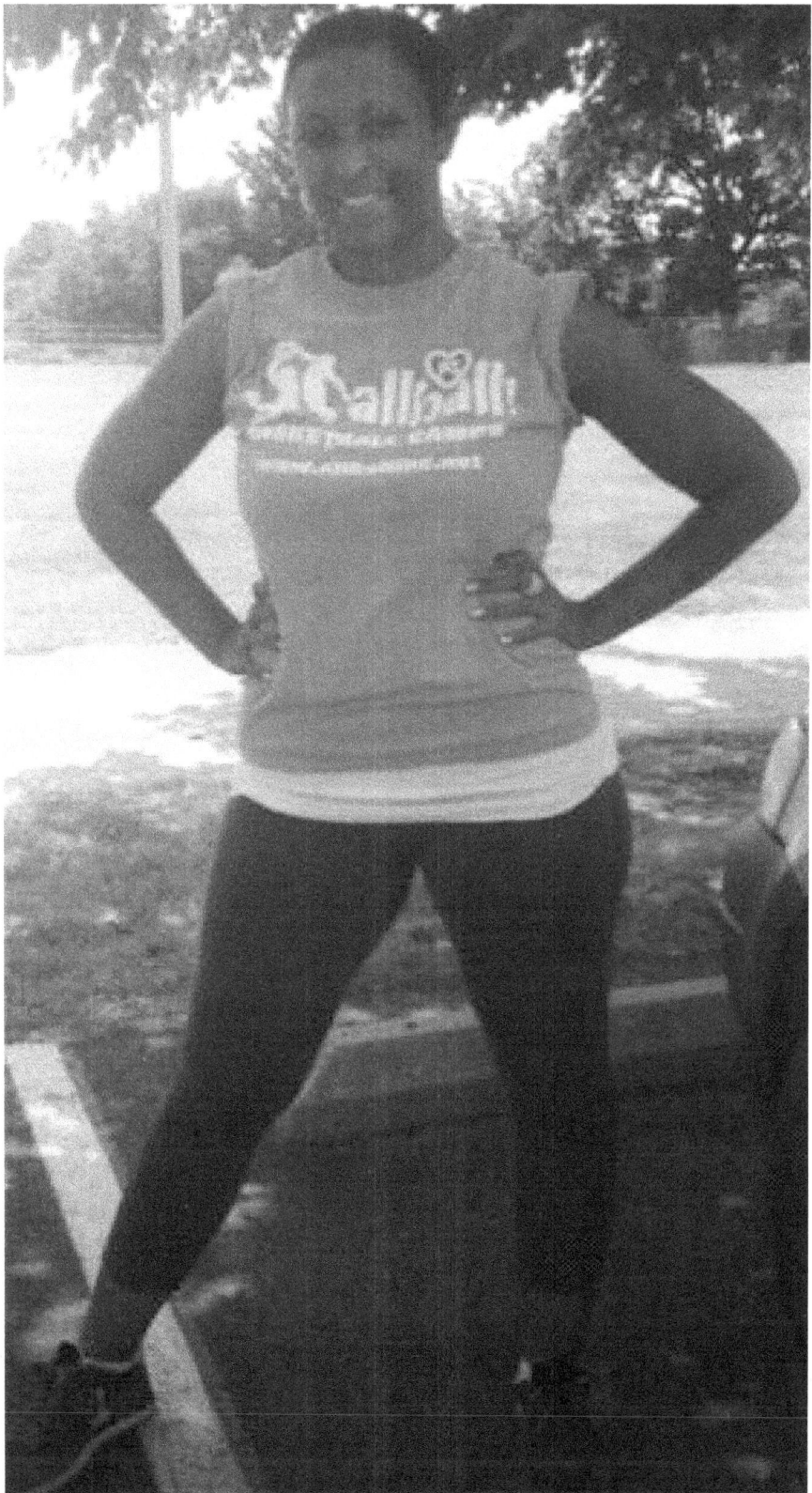

TAKING MY LIFE BACK

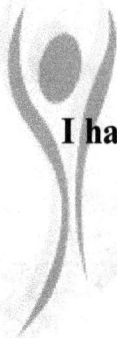

I have a renewed sense of purpose
and increased self-esteem.

YVONNE GRAY-WINKFIELD

TAKING MY LIFE BACK

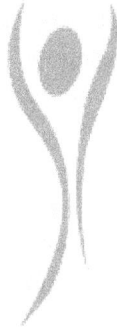

It gives me great pleasure and joy to share a piece of my journey about my struggle and fight to win the fight against obesity. It has been a twenty-one year battle, but I'm there! Phil 4:13 tells me I can do all things! Thank You Lord! I have tried many diets, weight loss products, programs and studies in the last 21 years. With all of them I have lost and regained the weight back, and some.

Over the last several years I have experienced quite a few losses that hit me pretty hard. I lost my father. Then, my mother was diagnosed with Dementia and she has been placed in a Senior Home (I'm her primary caregiver). My Mother-In-Law was the most recent loss in my life as for parental figures. As if that wasn't enough, I also lost my baby girl in a car accident at 18 years of age and then my baby brother whom I shared a very special relationship with passed away.

My health has had its ups and downs. Approximately 10 years ago, I was diagnosed with Thyroid Disease and was placed on medication. During which time, I began losing my hair and had to wear hair extensions to cover it up. Needless to say, this took a toll on me. I started looking for relief to help with the pain and losses. I turned to food, making it my comforter. I reached my highest weight of 262lbs in January 2012. I tried on a bathing suit for a trip and knew then it was time to take my life back.

I always shared with my daughter's my pain and sadness of trying to overcome this problem. My daughter Nakia told me to come to her home and she would help me get started on my road to fighting obesity. We set a date and she made a plan for me to follow. She took me to the supermarket and showed me what I should be eating. She told me to never leave home without my lunch bag. She said to control what you can and don't worry about the external foods unless you don't have your bag. Try to eat 75/25: 75% of what I cooked and 25% of foods from outside. I checked in with her from time to time and she finally pushed me past my fears of getting active and told me about a group called Black Girls Run (BGR)!

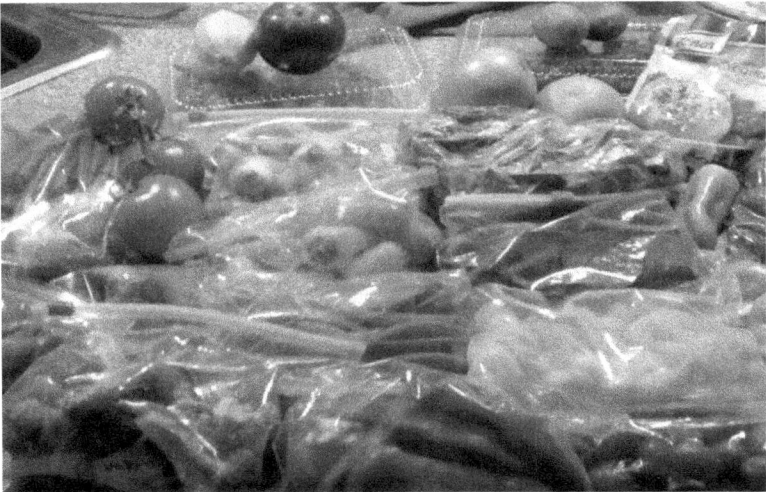

BGR has been such a supportive, inspiring and dedicated group of women who have given me courage to win this race! I felt at home from the start with many young and older women like myself fighting to take their control of their lives.

MOVEMENT IS MEDICINE

I began walking, then running side by side with my daughter Nakia. She would say, "Come on Mom, you can do it! Keep going!" It has been amazing! I would have never thought that at age 58, that I would be walking, jogging, wogging (a combination of walking and jogging) and entering races with my daughter. She has been a very inspirational to me. She has helped me to stay balanced and focused on fighting one round at a time. I have a renewed sense of purpose and increased self-esteemed.

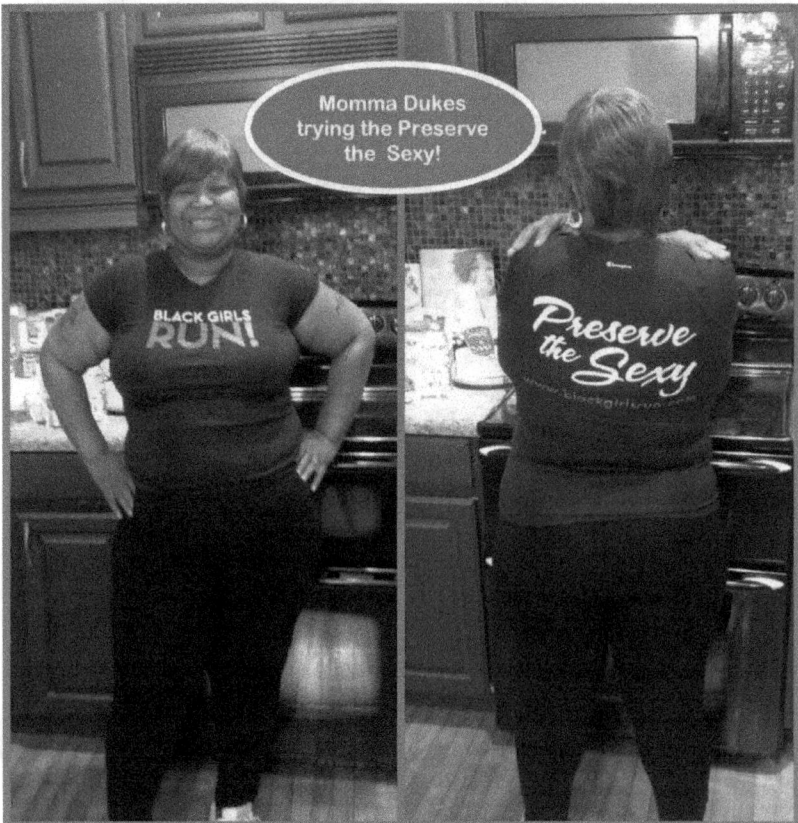

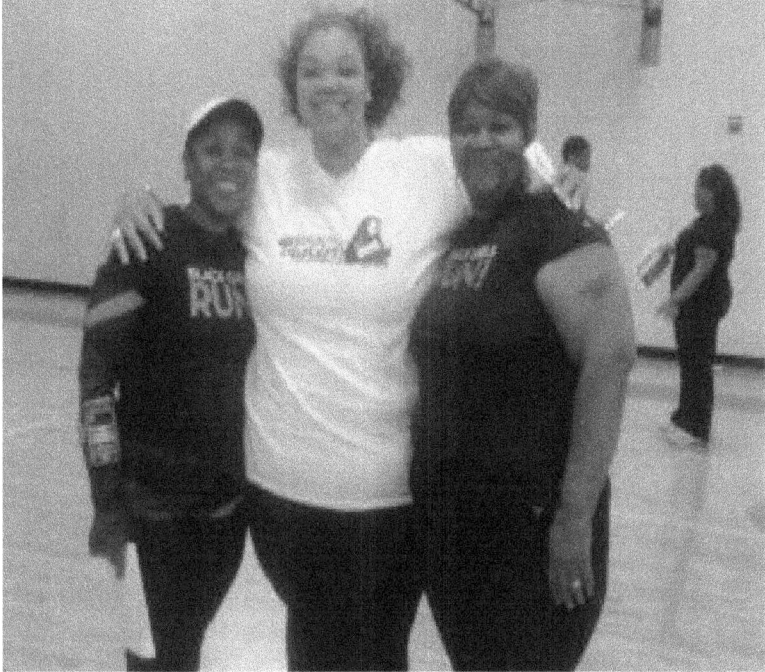

Since 1/31/12, I have lost 31pounds and several inches. I believe that life goes on even when we don't want it to. I have many goals now, but my most recent one is to lose thirty more pounds by my 58th birthday.

Enclosed are a few of my before & after photos. I feel better now than I have in a very long time. Things have also changed between my husband & I.

Smile,

Yvonne Gray-Winkfield (Aka Momma Dukes)

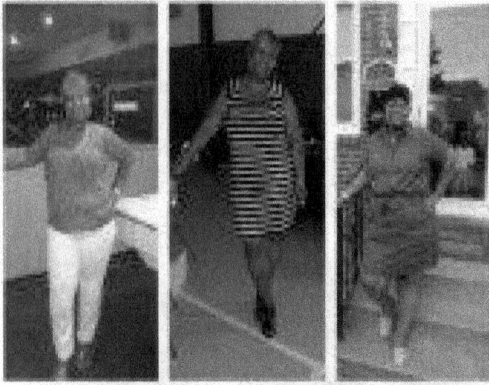

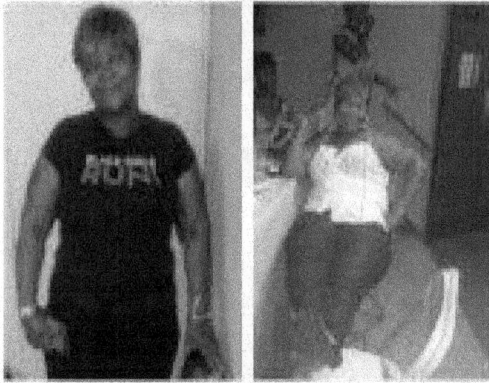

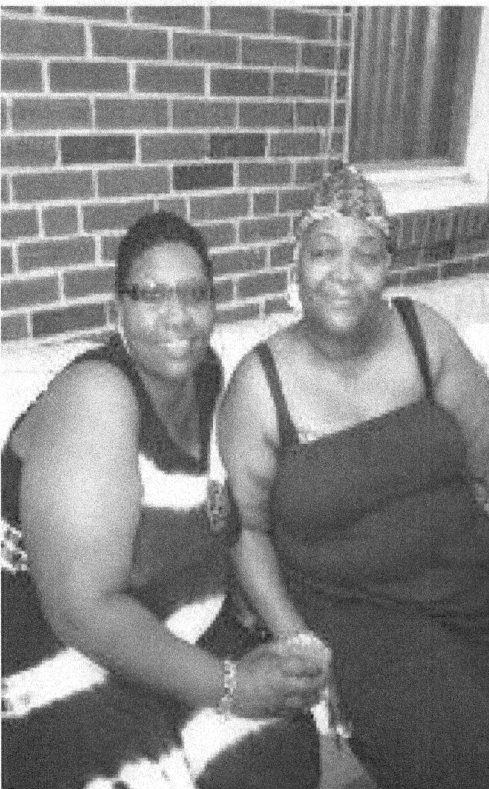

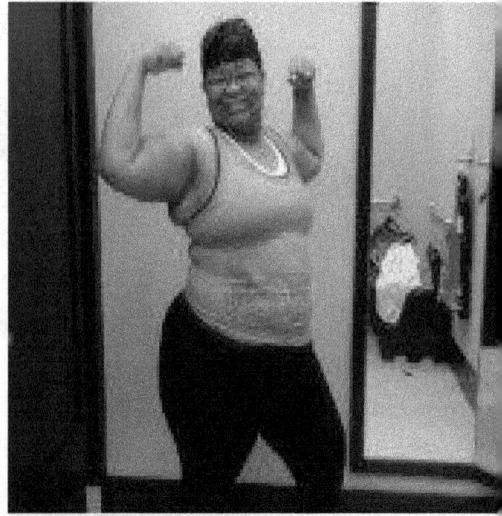

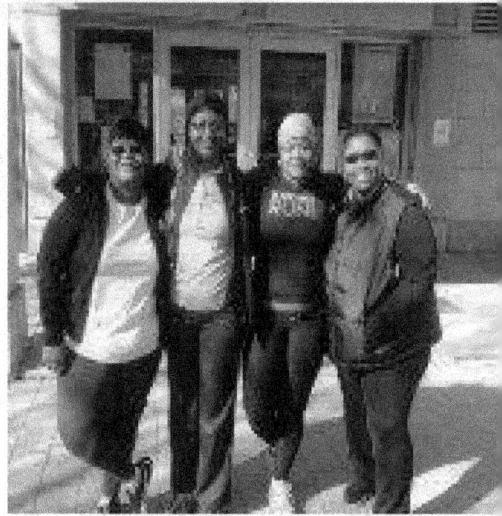

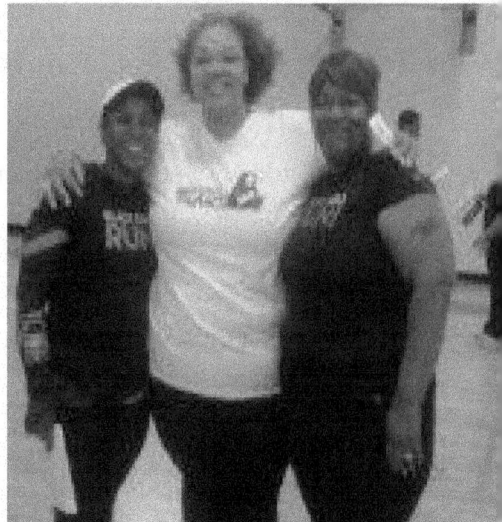

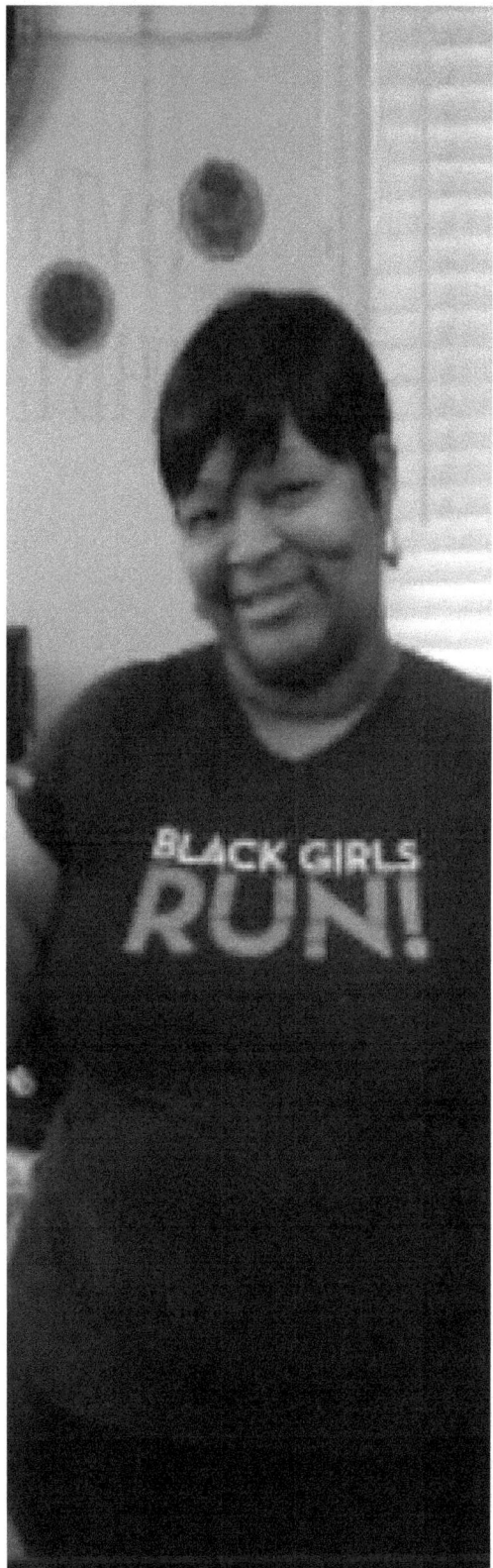
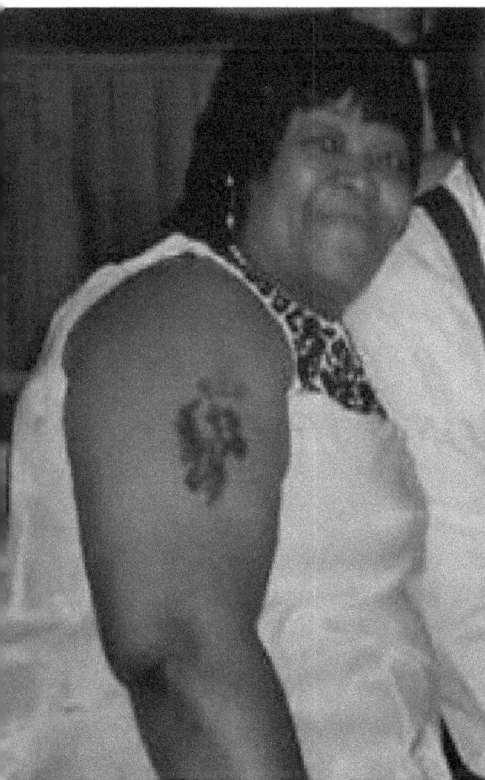

LOVING ME
FROM THE INSIDE OUT

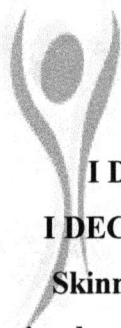

I DECIDED not to give up on me again.
I DECIDED that I wanted to **LOOK** how I felt.
Skinny is not my goal, but healthy and happy
is where I want to be as I continue my adventures.

SHIRELLE DIAMOND HOGANS

LOVING ME
FROM THE INSIDE OUT

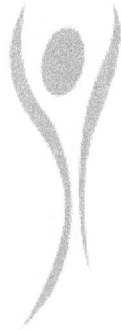

No one ever asks you how you feel. They only compliment you on how you look, or an item you are wearing. Never knowing the heavy weight fight you just had with yourself to find something that looked right, hung right and felt right. They weren't sitting courtside as you transformed into a meat packer and struggled, almost died, getting into a girdle. Their ears are deaf to the five alarm fire going on around your navel area because the top of your jeans are digging into your flesh.

MOVEMENT IS MEDICINE

I've often wanted to get a restraining order for my thighs to separate and stay in neutral corners. I've made numerous jokes about smelling bacon because I was sweating profusely. I laugh to ease my pain. I cry when no one is watching. Getting dressed is an adventure. Trying to maneuver the hardware when I have to use the bathroom belongs in RIPLEY'S BELIEVE IT OR NOT. One day I am going to write to the Guinness Book of World Records and enter "THICK GIRL UNDRESSING TO USE BATHROOM" as a category.

I've committed murder in my mind numerous times. I often mentally start choking people when they say, "You dress nice for a big girl." Really? Was the "BIG girl" part necessary? Did they just compliment me and insult me in the same breath? Why did my ability to be runway ready have to be limited to the big girl society? I love fashion. Shoes are my passion, and baby can I catwalk in my 6 inch heels! I know I can put an ensemble together, although it usually is an exhausting process, ending with all my clothes on the floor and me vowing to do something about my weight. SOON.

LOVING ME FROM THE INSIDE OUT

For years, I've never allowed people to take pictures of me from the side, only face shots, never full body. I didn't want to see "all of that", so I was bent on people not having evidence on how "big" I was. I limited myself to a pretty smile and fashion sense. When I walked into a room, I immediately scanned it, scoping out where to sit so no one had a full view of my spillage. I mastered how to speak in front of people while sucking it in and still breathing. The plan was to do it naturally and not look like I was in trauma. I was a moving target, a midget ninja in stilettos. I walk around and talk with my hands so that people are distracted on what I am saying, minimizing their assessment time of what I look like.

I've been the chubby girl for as long as I can remember. Middle school was barely tolerable, high school was a nightmare. As an adolescent I was molested by family members and felt abandoned and neglected in my own home. I didn't feel like anyone cared or loved me other than a service I provided. I am the oldest of four and as you can imagine, that came with a lot of responsibilities. As a teenager, the molestations continued and eventually I was brutally raped by a family member whom I later discovered was not related to me. I was a very intelligent young girl; Honor Society, High IQ club, Math Wiz, and I even participated in Shakespeare Competitions. None of that seemed to matter to anyone. Eventually I allowed all of that to slip away and allowed food and men to comfort me.

My heart is full of compassion for people. It's the main reason I became a Licensed Nurse. With all of my accomplishments, one would think that I didn't have a care in the world. They would be wrong. Childhood issues haunted me in my sleep. My nightmares carried into my awakened hours and I constantly second guessed myself. As a young adult, I now battled with domestic violence relationships and multiple miscarriages. I was always trying to please people, hoping they would love me. Most of the time, I would settle for them at least liking me. When all else failed, food and men where there. When the men disappeared, food had to put in overtime. It didn't have an opinion and it couldn't say no. As long as I had money and access to it, it was my slave and had to do what I told it to do, comfort me.

LOVING ME FROM THE INSIDE OUT

I have always been an outgoing person, traveling and finding fun things to do. I can use my son as a reason, however, I just like to have fun and often dragged him along. I have a reputation of being overzealous. At 35 years old, I have finally tapped into my adventurous side. It started a few years ago, after being dumped by a man and this time, even food let me down. A friend of mine asked me to walk around the athletic field with her so that we could talk.

Battling depression and thoughts of suicide, in addition to losing a man AND now food, of all times to bail on me, wasn't enough. I decided, why not?

At the time I wasn't saved, I actually didn't believe in God at all because of all of the horrific things I encountered in my life. My friend is a Bishop's daughter and could sing. We met on the condition that I did not want to discuss what I was going through and feeling. She agreed and did most of the talking, eventually making me laugh. Walking, laughing and her singing eventually cleared my head and allowed me to simply breathe. It was as if a weight had been lifted off my shoulders. At the conclusion of our walk, I could think clearer and had a different perspective of my current situation. *Food was spared my angry wrath and walking became my solace.*

I join a gym every now and then when my finances can handle it. I now enjoy, and may I add ROCK OUT, in zumba, line dancing, kickboxing and lifting weights. I have a wild side and have recently enjoyed Rock Climbing and riding the Mechanical Bull. Jetskiing and parasailing are on my 'to do' list, I'm making time to create the opportunity. Not to mention I have a teenage son now that I enjoy spending time with. We run suicides together, play basketball and laser tag. Let him tell it, I do way too much for a "mom". Even with all my excitement and adventures, I wasn't happy. Busy yes, active yes, but not happy.

Battling my weight for years with exercise here and there wasn't working anymore. I got fed up with just maintaining a weight that wasn't healthy anyway. All my girdles seemed to have a short life expectancy. I hated looking in the mirror more and more. I finally got a glimpse of me from the side and was horrified that everyone else had already seen my dysfunction. Ironic that my first thought was about what everyone else had seen and not that this was actually *my body*. I realized then, my problem of pleasing people and lack of self value still dwelled within me.

I've cried numerous times in disbelief that I allowed myself to get here. The people I was trying to please didn't have to live in this body, I did. So why didn't I love myself enough to change it versus just dressing it up to look presentable? I wasn't ready to answer these questions. I ran from them, as always, straight to my potato chip bag. I am a salt fanatic. Cakes, pies and cookies can't please me like a bag of chips or a sandwich can. While attempting to get my comfort food, I suddenly stopped. This was the problem. If I didn't do something about it quick, my son wouldn't have a mother anymore. That's the thought that started me on my journey of loving me from the inside out. Eventually, as much as I love and adore my son, not only did I need to be there for him, I decided I was going to be there for **me**!

I realized that although I had moved on, I was letting the past control me. My mental immobility was blowing me up like a helium balloon and I was literally bursting at the seams.

Jeans that were once loose on me became tighter. Shirts were bulging, threatening to put someone's eye out if a button popped off. I made several excuses of what was happening. I conjured up excuses like: my clothes shrunk, I'm retaining water and my doctors 2 all time favorites: I have Ascites (fluid in my abdomen) or PCOS (cysts on my ovaries, which can cause weight gain). I had my doctor do a full blood panel workup. I couldn't fool myself anymore. My finances forced me to evict myself from my mentally dysfunctional 24hr shack of food heaven. I couldn't and wouldn't buy one more piece of clothing to hide my shame. I stood in front of the mirror, got naked, pulled out my camera and started taking pictures.

I look at the pictures almost every day. No matter what I wore or how creative I was at covering up, my pictures spoke a thousand words of dysfunction. Don't get me wrong, I say nice things about myself all the time and I know I have many beautiful characteristics about me, but I also had to force myself to look at myself entirely. It was time to move. Move from despair and heartache to a place of peace and joy. Move from camouflaging my lack of self love to embracing the diva I feel I am on the inside of me. My mental movement ignited a fire in me to put plans in place.

I worked out at the gym as much as I could. I learned to love the elliptical machine, it's my favorite. When my finances started becoming questionable, I took my determination to the streets. I found a track and a park that I could work-out on for free. My music playlist pushes and encourages me. I started off just walking but got bored. I love a challenge so I started running the inclines. When that became easier, I included running up and down the steps, like I was Rocky Balboa. I even created my own meet-up in Philly to race up and down the Rocky steps at the monument.

As I stated before, I laugh to ease my pain. One day as I was running with my son, whom encourages and celebrates me as well, I heard this popping noise. The faster I ran, the louder and faster it got. Imagine the mixed tears of frustration and amusement when we discovered it was my lower stomach hitting my upper thighs as I ran!!! My son didn't know whether to laugh or hug me. Now, I believe, you really aren't getting a good work out until your stomach and thighs start clapping for you!

MOVEMENT IS MEDICINE

I tried to stay creative because boredom will kill my passion.

I started participating in races such as: Cerebral Palsy walk in Philadelphia, Aids walk in Delaware and the Domestic Violence Walk in Delaware. I've run a little and walked the majority of the races. I pat myself on the back because I not only tried but I completed them and I have the pictures to prove it!

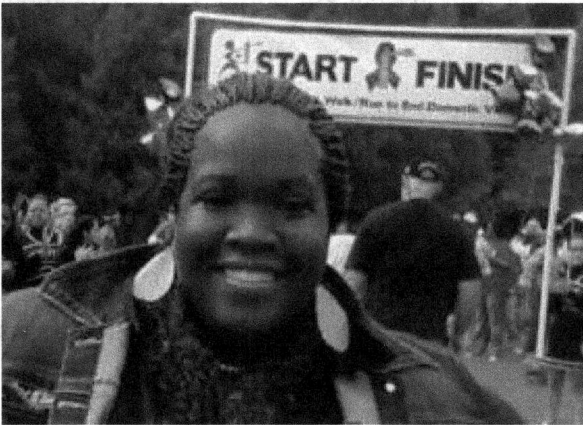

My weight would go up and down a few pounds because I was active, but I never saw a significant decline. Discouraged, I started seeing a "weight doctor" that I heard other women were visiting. As long as I had money, I lost weight. I would pay to take appetite suppressant pills, water pills and a vitamin shot. When the money ran out, I would maintain that weight and eventually it would start rising again, despite my sporadic adventures and exercise. Frustrated and about to knock on depressions door and ask for some salt and sugar, I started talking to the Nutritionist at my place of employment.

I have issues being vulnerable. I don't mind telling people the fluff and surface things, or even the hard issues that I've overcome. However, being vulnerable and exposed to people, especially people I don't have a history with, about my current issues are hard for me. Heidi, the Nutritionist, was very sincere and helpful. She told me I needed to change my eating habits in addition to working out. She also told me I needed to be consistent and monitor how I felt when I ate. She weighed me every week and tracked my progress. She was hard on me when I needed her to be, but she also celebrated me like crazy when I was making progress.

For the most part, I have changed my eating habits. Although I still splurge occasionally, I don't do it as often as I used to. I chose to love me from the inside out and I refuse to go back to killing myself slowly. I have always taken pictures. I love being able to track my family's journey. Pictures tell stories and trigger memories. Pictures, for me, help me create a new and happy life. One I didn't have as a child. I have my moments of sadness and depression is always eager and ready to come over for a visit. Instead of food, I try to exercise to clear my head. Prayer, laughing and looking at pictures are also part of my "GET IT TOGETHER QUICK BEFORE YOU LOSE IT" techniques.

I decided not to give up on me again. I decided that I wanted to LOOK how I felt. Skinny is not my goal, but healthy and happy is where I want to be as I continue my adventures. I am on my own journey of loving me from the inside out and this time; walking, crawling, laughing, kicking and screaming through the pain…I am going to get it done. I often run now because I can and love to see the look of shock on others faces as I pass them. I am not a fan of running per say. However, I am proud to say that I finally became a fan of me.

Look for me on the beach doing my Baywatch run, while I'm this size as well as when I reach my goal look :)

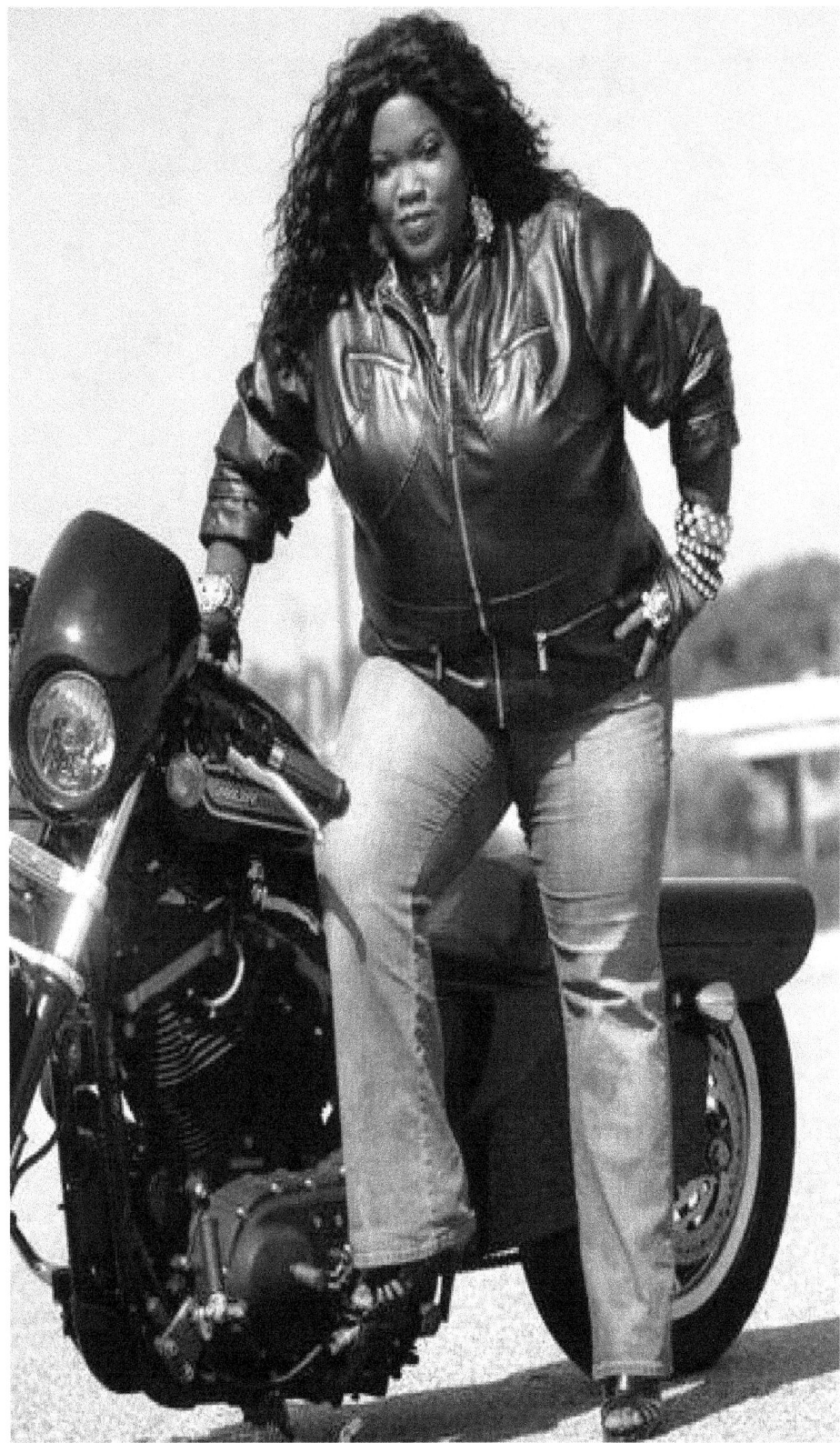

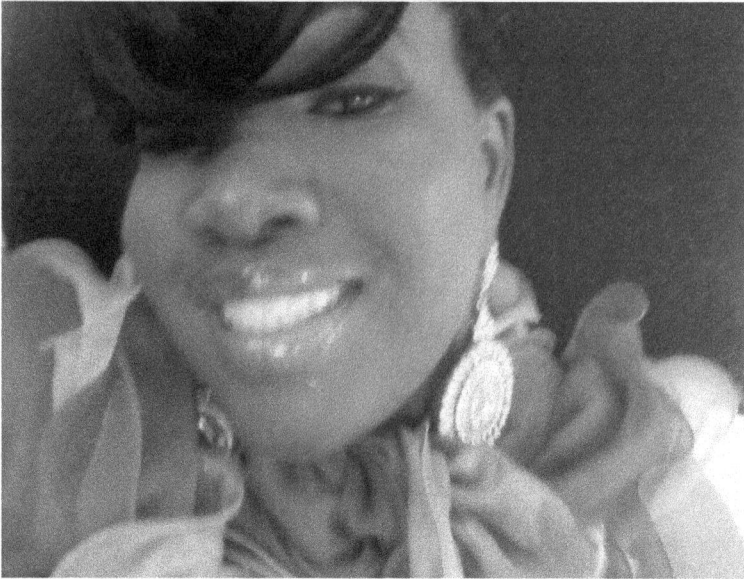

Shirelle DIAMOND Hogans is an Empowerment Speaker and CEO of DIAMOND'S WORLD INC. She is also the Creative Empress of RADIKAL PUBLICATIONS, an Author, Actress, Licensed Nurse, Licensed Minister of the Gospel and mother of one incredible son.

Nothing excites her more than encouraging people to fulfill their destiny. She is always in the mood for a challenge, adventure and a photo shoot. Her smile and passion are contagious.

Visit Diamond and Diamond's World Inc at:
www.diamonds-world.org

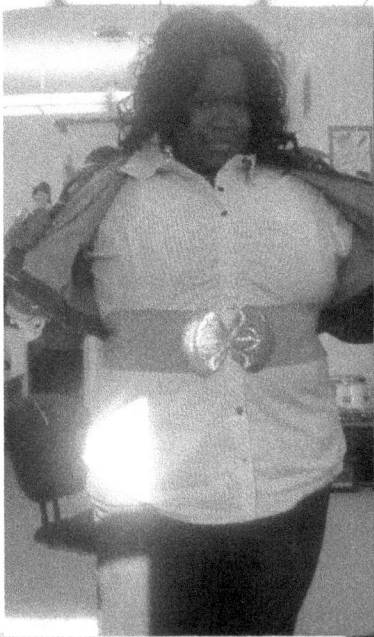

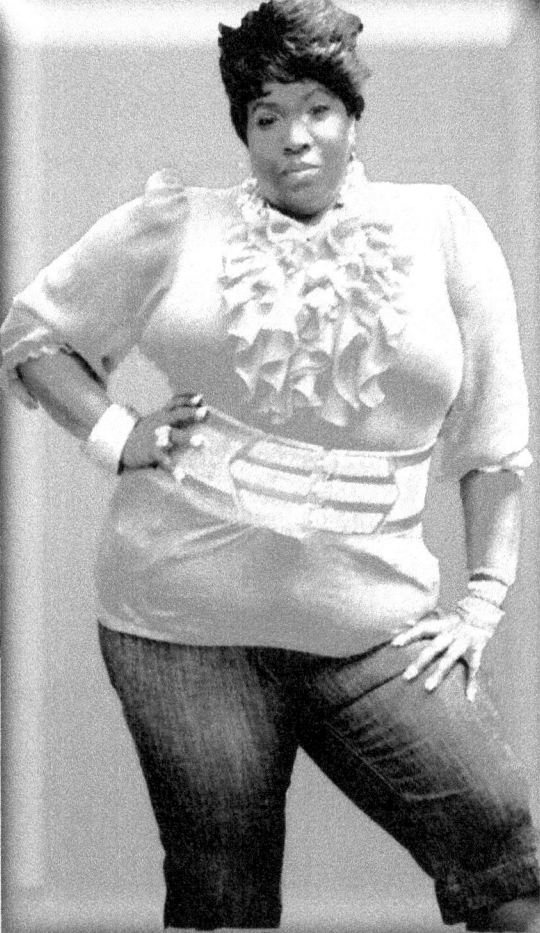

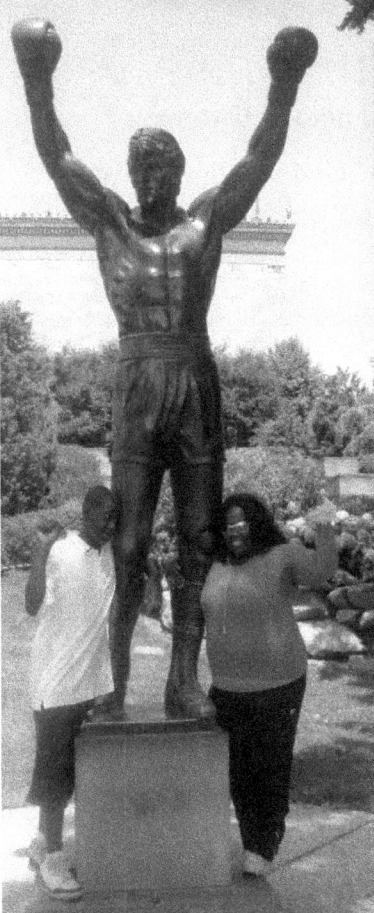

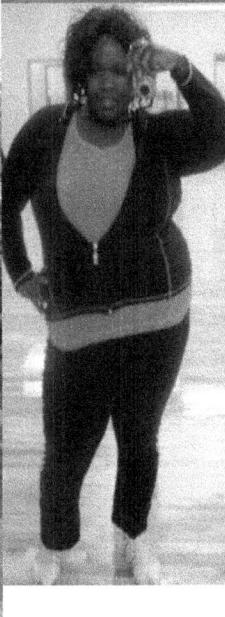

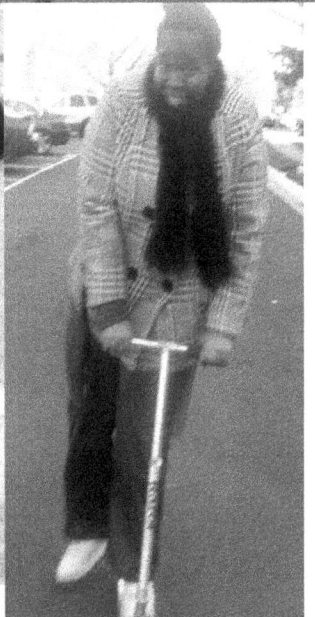

THE DISCOVERY OF ME

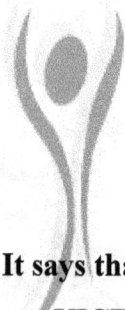

I MATTER.

I have PURPOSE.

It says that I am the top and not the bottom.

That I am VICTORIOUS, and that God will fight for me.

E. PATRICE THREADGILL

THE DISCOVERY
OF ME

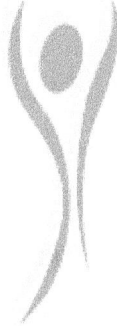

I'm a little embarrassed to tell you that despite my wonderful childhood, I lived it not knowing who I was. I lived in the expectations of my parents, my friends, church folk, and my former husband. This is the thing that has stunted my personal growth in my adult years. My movement journey was and still is; the discovery of me, my identity, my purpose, and living the life God intended me to have.

I was the only daughter and the youngest in my family. I was also a preacher's kid (PK), which basically means that I shared my parents with the church. While this opportunity did afford me more sisterhood and "cousin" relationships, I do feel in retrospect, that I missed having my mom and dad to myself. Because people knew me as the "Reverend's daughter", that was who I was entirely. I felt like I was somebody simply because he was somebody.

With my peers, I struggled. I had a few strikes against me, I thought. I was definitely not part of the "in" crowd. To be popular, back then, meant to be shapely, light-skinned, and "good hair". I was that skinny, dark-complexioned girl, whose hair wafted of Sulfur 8 on the playground at recess. When it came to boys, my friends got notes passed in class, I did not. At least not from the boys I would have liked to receive notes from. I felt like I wasn't pretty enough.

On top of everything else, I was teased as a child. My mom named me after her mother, Elva. She told me that my name was beautiful and that she thought Elva Patrice sounded like a movie star. For me, it was an unending opportunity for those who knew to burst into every Elvis Presley rendition, with lips and gyration included. El-Vi-Ra, was the other popular diddy. I used to cry and became ashamed of my name, so I hid it, in order to shield myself of the torment it evoked. I embraced my nickname, not because I liked it, but because it was better than Elva.

I later realized that I did not embrace my own self because others did not embrace me. I had allowed other people and their opinions to dictate my feelings, my thoughts, and my actions. It did not seem to matter to them, that it hurt my feelings, so I learned to stifle my feelings, conform and even laugh with them when I was teased. It seemed to end a lot sooner if I gave in. The fight for myself was leaving me. I ate and swallowed my hurt emotionally because I felt no one seemed to care.

This unsure 19 year old married and added three more titles to her life to juggle. I became a wife, mother, and preacher's wife. I tried to fill these roles as I had seen my mother do. I was committed to a dysfunctional relationship. The main dysfunction was my own because I had not known myself, and did not bring her to the table. I sacrificed my "life" to be what others needed me to be. Somewhere in the middle, I began dying from the inside out. The truth of the matter is, how could I expect someone to love me, when they could not see me?

MOVEMENT IS MEDICINE

I was a stay-at-home mom, which I absolutely enjoyed. Although my 3 daughters were very close in age, the joy of being their mom was easy to get lost in. I did not realize it, but I now know that God was beginning to teach me how to take care of myself. I began to work out with a program that came on TV daily. I found that it was a good stress reliever, and I was able to manage myself better. Cardio became my friend that I enjoyed each day. It allowed my body to work in such a way that my mind was able to settle. I could then read my bible, pray and make better decisions.

I loved God from an early age, and wanted to please Him. I understood His sacrifice for my sin, and tried to live a sacrificial life of dying on the inside to identify with Him. I did not understand that He wanted me to give myself to Him. That He wanted to bless me and live an abundant life here on Earth. I tried my best to conform to the BE-attitudes, even though people took advantage of me, hurt me, and used me. I kept telling myself to be kind to my enemies, love those who persecute me, forgive those who hurt me. These were things God wanted me to do, but not in my own strength, but in Him and through Him. I considered myself a sufferer for the cause of Jesus Christ.

THE DISCOVERY OF ME

I believe the breaking point for me was the deterioration of my marriage, my house was in foreclosure, and no provision had been made for our family's future. If ever there was a bottom, this was it. I went into the "survival mode" that the Lord had taught me. I began seeking Him in the morning through prayer and meditation in His word. This set a covering over my mind. It gave me something, other than the stressors, to think about while at work.

I went to the gym and worked out every day. That allowed me to release the stress that was building up in my body. Stress will kill you, if you let it. I ate well. Organic meats, whole grains, things that came from the ground. This blocked the lethargic, depressed feeling that can overwhelm you after eating poorly. Lastly, I went to bed early. I made a worship CD and set it on repeat to play quietly all night. I charged the atmosphere of my bedroom into the throne room of God, and my spirit worshipped all night long. I did not realize what I was doing at the time, but I was disarming the devil of opportunities to speak negativity into my spirit. God carried me through what should have been the worst time of my life.

My spirit opened up in such a way that I had never experienced God before. He began to reveal His deep love and concern for me. He cared about the details of my life. He told me how He was going to heal my hurts and He wanted me whole. He challenged me to trust Him, to stop listening to everybody's voice and opinion, and seek Him only.

He gave me my life's verse, (Jeremiah 29:11)" For I know the plans I have for you," declares the LORD, "plans to prosper you and not to harm you, plans to give you hope and a future." After that revelation set in, God opened up the windows of my mind and my life and blew fresh air into me. He began, and still is cleaning the cobwebs of my past, so that they don't dictate my future.

I am still in the act of "becoming", becoming who God created me to be. I am still learning how to become comfortable with myself, whether people like it or not. I respect their opinion, but they don't determine my direction, God does.

THE DISCOVERY OF ME

I now embrace my name, I am Elva Patrice Threadgill. Elva means, "a ripple in the stream".

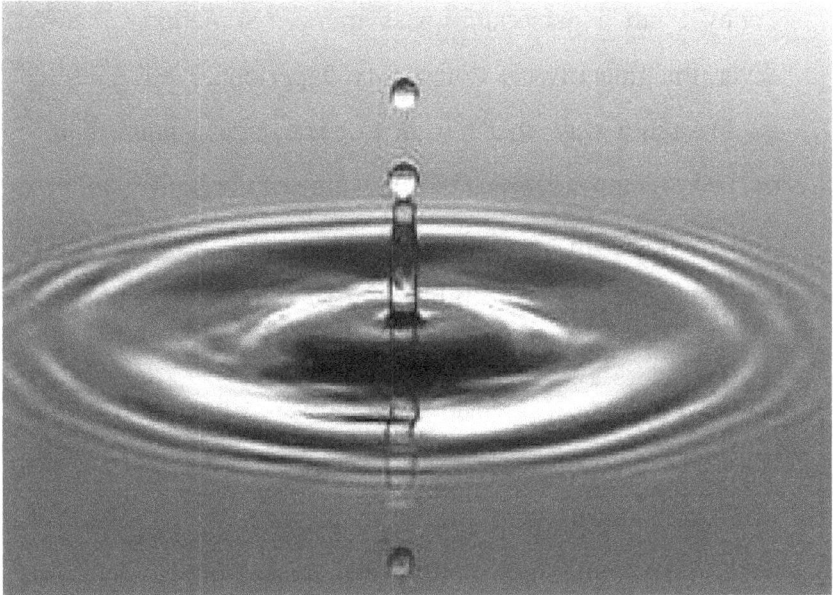

That means I MATTER.

I have PURPOSE.

It says that I am the top and not the bottom.

That I am VICTORIOUS, and that God will fight for me.

He wants me to live transparent so the world can see Him in me. No longer hiding or wearing masks, pretending I am someone I am not.

Today I am a personal fitness trainer. Something I could never imagine myself doing. My experiences have altered me in such a way, that I want to encourage women. I have learned and am still learning: the value of the body, soul, and spirit connection. We as women tend to neglect ourselves because the responsibilities of parenting, finances, relationships, and sometimes church responsibilities, seem to scream the loudest. I desire to empower women that we are worth the investment of exercise, and to honor their bodies with good nutrition to fuel it to perform their daily tasks well. They will feel better, and make better decisions because of those two components alone.

I want to encourage you, my sister to love who you are. You are fearfully and wonderfully made. Your life has meaning and God has purpose for every experience you have had. You can move forward from where you are today. Those dreams and desires inside of you, God put them there.

THE DISCOVERY OF ME

I encourage you to live in harmony with yourself first. Be true to yourself. What you think, what you say, and what you do, expresses to yourself and the world who you really are.

When you do these things, they validate your own voice, opinion, and self-worth. Nobody can do that for you. You may encounter many negative people that will laugh at or discourage your dreams and visions. That is okay. Don't become defensive, it's okay. They are not you, nor can you expect them to think like you.

Embrace your authentic self. Bloom where you are planted and make a difference. I challenge you to move forward in your thought life, because if you change your thinking, you will change your life. Dream in color and write your vision on paper. You can do whatever you put your mind to, it is never too late. Things don't change overnight, but little by little, small successes add up to huge victories!

Be encouraged! You are fearfully and wonderfully made. You were made in the image of God Himself! He has a wonderful purpose for your life, run after it. You can do it!! You have a crowd of witnesses in this book celebrating you and cheering you on to success. God bless.

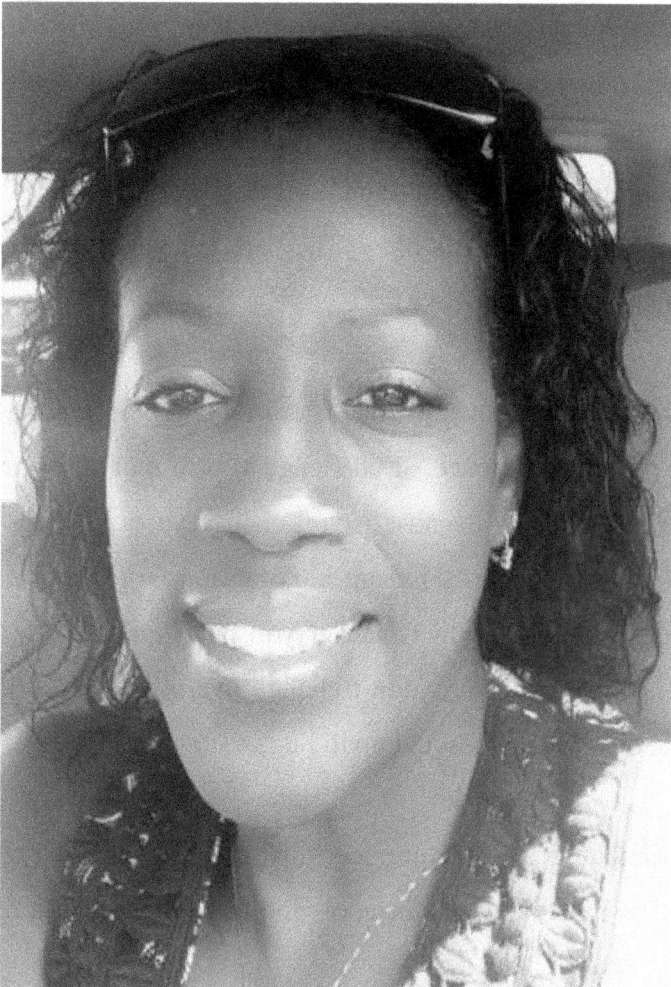

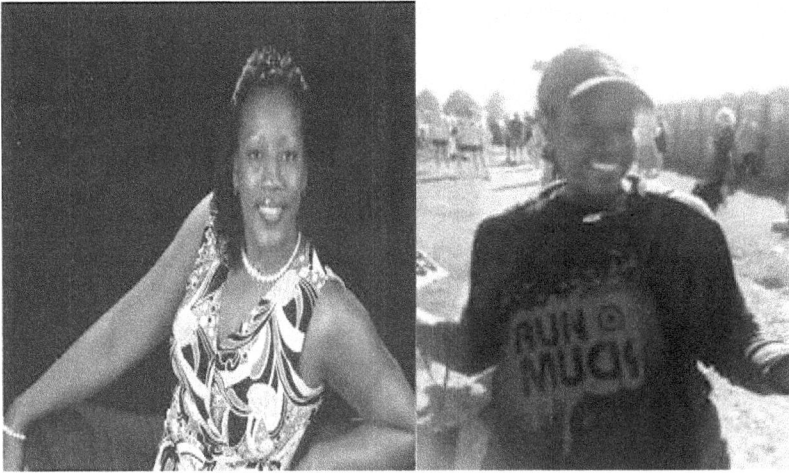

E. Patrice Threadgill is a current resident of Edgewater Park, New Jersey. She is a wife and the mother of 3 daughters, has a son-in-love, and a son by marriage. She is the proud grandmother of 5 amazing grandchildren. She works full-time for the State of New Jersey, and part-time as a Certified Personal Fitness Trainer.

She is also a Certified Christian Counselor, certified by the America Association of Christian Counselors (AACC). Her life goal is to motivate, encourage, and empower women to pursue their dreams, to be healthy from the inside out, and to live in the abundance God has for us all. Her life verse is Jeremiah 29:11"For I know the plans I have for you," declares the LORD, "plans to prosper you and not to harm you, plans to give you hope and a future."

SEXY BEFORE, SEXIER AFTER

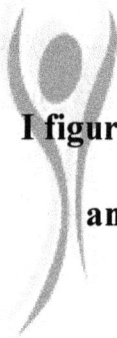

I figure no one else is going to love me
like I could love myself
and I love me a whole bunch!

TAMMI WILLIAMS JORDAN

SEXY BEFORE, SEXIER AFTER

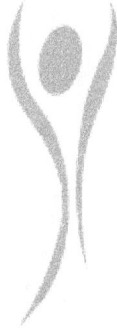

My journey, my journey, my journey? Oh my goodness, what did I get myself into? Where do I begin? Why am I doing this? I'm doing this because Movement Is Medicine. I'm doing this because my sista friend, my sister in Christ, my sister of the Ville thought enough of me to ask me to be involved. I'm doing this because God gave me the courage and the determination to want to do better.

I'm 42, (I can't believe I just put my business "out on the street" like that), 5'11", and had been approximately 260 lbs for as long as I can remember. My self esteem is great! In fact some think I border on vanity. I figure no one else is going to love me like I could love myself and I love me a whole bunch! I knew that I was overweight, but my attitude was, "So what, I'm still sexy!"

Several months ago, Mona started posting daily updates regarding her journey to be healthy. As I read her updates and watched her metamorphis, I became more and more excited for her. As my excitement for her grew, my personal desire to be healthy developed.

On June 18, 2012, I woke up at 5:00 am as I usually do, but this time it was my first official day of summer vacation. I could have rolled over and went back to sleep but I thought of Mona and said to myself, "If she can do it, so can I!" I climbed out of the bed, washed up, put on my shorts and sneakers and walked to the park a few blocks from my home. At the park, I walked the path 4 times because someone told me it was the equivalent of a mile. After the fourth lap, I returned home to drink water and rest. It was exhausting, but I felt great!

SEXY BEFORE, SEXIER AFTER

Guess what? The next day at 5 am, the alarm went off and I got up and walked. I did it again the day after that and the day after that! Two months later, I'm walking approximately 3 miles several times a week. Some days, I fall off the wagon, but my sistas encourage me by posting their own journeys on FaceBook. My husband tells me daily how proud he is of me. My doctor shares her own journey with me and even gave me a two week pass to a boxing class.

I really am not trying to lose weight. My goal is simply to be healthy. However, when I stepped on a scale a few weeks ago it said 242! If I thought I was sexy before…watch out!

Got to go now, I need to walk.

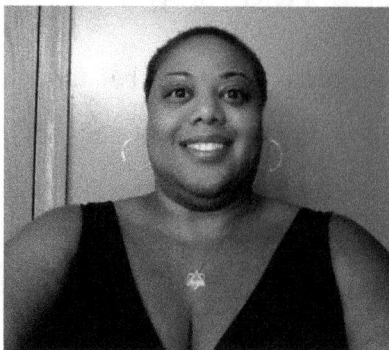

Originally born and reared *Tammi Williams Jordan* attended Millersville University of Pennsylvania where she earned a Bachelor of Arts in Social Work and a Master of Education in Counselor Education. Prior to becoming a licensed school counselor for Big Walnut City Schools in Sunbury Ohio, she was a Student Affairs Administrator at Capital University, a Counselor at Columbus State Community College, and an Educational Consultant for the Ohio Department of Education. Tammi is passionate about helping young people reach their highest academic, career, and personal goals and some days is even amazed that she is compensated for having "fun" all day. In her free time, you can find Tammi reading a good book, spending time with her grandchildren, or providing public service as a member of her sorority.

GET UP AND *MOVE* SOMETHING

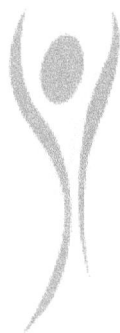

DEALING WITH MY PAIN
HEAD ON

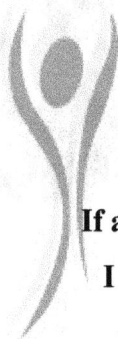

If and when I feel sad or depressed
I now know how to deal with it.
Instead of pills or food,
I run and create memories with my children.

RENEE SAMIYAH JOHNSON-RAMZIDDIN

DEALING WITH MY PAIN HEAD ON

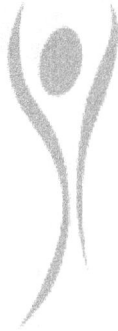

I never intended to share my journey with anyone outside my immediate family and close friends. I'm honored to share with a wonderful group of women and hope my journey can inspire others.

My journey, from childhood, consisted and started because of one reason, PAIN. Unable to deal with the pain and hurt, I went through life wondering why I behaved certain ways, questioned all my decisions, and never really understood the outcome of those decisions. The only coping skills I had were crying and eating!

My PAIN side swiped me back in 2006 when I had an anxiety attack. Days prior to the attack, I was driving home one evening and drove past a familiar area that gave me the chills. I pulled over to catch my breath and gather myself before I went any further. Still not knowing what just happened, I went home. My mind raced and I tried to sleep, but couldn't. I kept having these visuals and memories of my childhood. Days went by and I couldn't eat or sleep. One day at work, it happened again. Not only did I have an anxiety attack, I had an outer body experience. I literally felt like I stepped outside of my body and was looking at myself. I lost control of ME. All of a sudden these horrible memories of my childhood flooded in at once. I ran and locked myself in a bathroom stall. I began crying and ripping my clothes off. I was so hot, it felt as if I were in a sauna. I remember calling my mom trying to tell her what was happening and friends trying to come to my aid. The next thing I knew I was in the emergency room.

Once I finally came to, I was able to understand the events that took place. I suppressed all the horrible things that happened to me as a child, at the hands of my own father. I wasn't ready to talk to anyone about the events. The doctors gave me medication to help me sleep and sent me home. I still knew in the back of my mind I had to tell my family what was happening with me. I got up the courage to finally tell my mom that my dad, her husband, at the time, molested me from the age of 5 until 15.

Everyone had millions of questions, and honestly, I didn't know how to answer them. I tried to sleep, to not think about it but, that didn't work. My doctor suggested I go to a support group for victims of abuse. I joined the group but in my opinion it made it worse. After the group meeting, I went home and took some sleeping pills. I took more than what I was supposed to. *I JUST WANTED TO SLEEP AND NOT REMEMBER.*

The next thing I could remember was being in the emergency room. I had been involuntary committed (302'd) by my sister. While in the hospital I found out I was pregnant, which elevated things to a completely different level. I was admitted into a facility for about a week to learn how to release my thoughts and work through them. I was denied medicine due to my pregnancy so it was harder than I thought it would be. *The medication couldn't knock me out. I had to deal with my PAIN head on.*

I began to talk about some of the memories I kept envisioning. The more I expressed it, the more I started realizing a lot of the decisions I made in life stemmed from my abuse. The way I would always be in a boy's face or crossing that line of, "No, he is off limits because he is family." It's too many examples I can give to show all the mistakes I made growing up due to that man taking my childhood away from me. After the sessions were over, I was permitted to come home and start what they called *"A NEW WAY OF LIVING."*

I started seeing a psychologist who helped me understand my behaviors weren't my fault. The guilt I felt, from enjoying the touches my body felt as a child, wasn't my fault. How I let that man trick me into not telling anyone, or how once I suppressed those memories until I was an adult, wasn't my fault. None of it was my fault, but I still blamed myself for it all. Eating the pain away made it easy. I was pregnant, so I didn't care about gaining the weight, but in actuality, I was slipping into depression with every piece of food I put into my mouth. I stopped going to my sessions I basically shut down. I didn't want to talk about it anymore. I was convinced I was a "screwed-up-lost-cause", so what was the point. The statue of limitations had been surpassed and unfortunately, I couldn't press charges. Mentally I was lost. However, my unborn child helped take my mind off the memories. I knew I was carrying a baby that I was responsible for and had to do right my child. I started focusing on that and I felt better.

As time moved on, I still felt like something was wrong. Something was missing inside of me, but I wasn't sure what. I put on a mask in front of everyone so they would think I was fine, but I wasn't. I was stressed to the point that the last six months of my pregnancy was spent on bed rest. Finally, the day came and I had a healthy, happy baby girl. After giving birth, I wasn't concerned about losing weight. Anyone else would have been working to lose the weight, but not me. I ate from sun up to sun down. Food was my best friend. I would go to the doctors and see how much weight I gained and could care less. I was always out of breath walking up a flight of stairs, but I knew when I got to the top there was a snack waiting for me as a reward.

After all the eating and binging, it never occurred to me that I gained 23 lbs. I was in food heaven. One day my sister said, "You better slow down on your snacks." I thought, "What does she know?" I continued to eat. One day, I went to the doctor and told her I think I have asthma and my stomach kept giving me problems. She told me straight out, "You're not asthmatic, you're fat. You need to lose weight and soon!" That was definitely an eye opener. From that doctor visit on, I started eating better and walking. It was a struggle indeed, but I was doing okay.

I was doing well until 2008. Once again PAIN had snuck its way in. My 16 year old daughter, at the time, tried to hang herself. To walk in a room and see your child hanging in a closet is very traumatic, something I will never forget. While getting her the help she needed, I didn't realize I was binge eating yet again. It was the only way I could stay up and make sure she didn't try to hurt herself again. Before I knew it , the weight I lost was back. God blessed me to still have my daughter but blessed me with my bad habit as well.

DEALING WITH MY PAIN HEAD ON

It was recommended that we see a family counselor and I'm glad we did. She was definitely God sent. This woman helped me work through the traumatic events that occurred and made me realize what was ultimately missing in my life, affection towards my children. She helped me take back the power he took from me. I never realized until I sat down and talked to her, that he took not only from me but from my children too. They deserved a better mom! It was sad that I could show men affection better than I could show my children. Until this day I'm still learning to hug, kiss and tell my children I love them. Yes, my children know I love them, but now I wanted to show it.

Feeling better, I started walking with my sister, a mile here a mile there. Before I knew it, I was using exercise to release whatever stress I was dealing with. Instead of binge eating, I would run. I now have a different type of PAIN, runner's pain! However, a little stretching here and there takes care of that! I am down 17 pounds and still working hard to keep the weight off. Do I still snack? YES! However, I now know the importance of a good snack versus a bad snack. Running saved my life. My Black Girls Run (BGR) partners nicknamed me "Smiley" because I refuse to fall back into the depressed state I was in for all those years. I always have a know how to deal with it. Instead of pills or food, I run and create memories with my children.

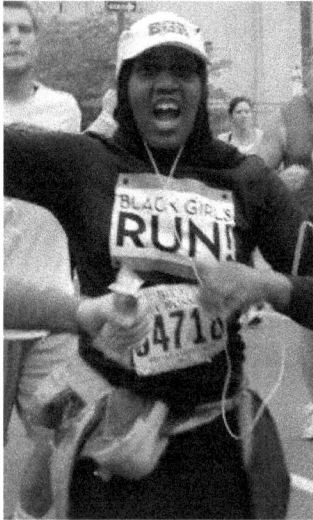

Renee is a 39 years old wife of three years, mother of ten blended children and also a grandmother. Despite my obstacles, I still find the time and strength to focus on my goals. When I first got into my stress release therapy, I was just walking. I never intended to enter into any races. Since then, I have completed "The Broad Street Run" twice which is a ten mile run.

Thanks to my support team BGR (Black Girls Run). I have been in other races for different cures, 5ks as well as 8ks. In total I have three medals and still on my way to more. My biggest accomplishment will be finishing my first Half Marathon in October.

I thank God everyday for giving me the best support system I could ever ask for, family and friends. When I joined BGR, I was scared being the only Muslim female out there. However, these ladies opened their arms and hearts to me. Yes, I get stares when I'm out there being covered and running, but my BGR sisters always have my back. Without Allah, family and friends I wouldn't be able to push like I do or have the courage to share my journey with you.

THE COURAGE TO START AGAIN

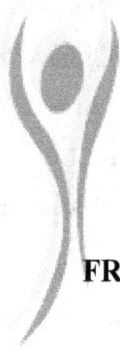

FREE from pain,

FREE from suffering,

FREE from self pity,

FREE to gain my life back,

FREE to be a warrior,

FREE to be available for greatness.

NAKIA HENDERSON

THE COURAGE
TO START AGAIN

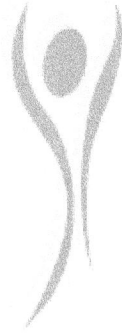

I remember crying in the shower one day in December 2010 and saying to God, "I have done all that I can do, I surrender to you." At that moment, nothing happened. However today, I am a firm believer that He heard my cry.

Over the past few years, I have experienced several tragedies, losses, and disappointments. I had learned to live with them until it all became too hard to live "there" anymore. I had to change. I have gone from victim, to victor, to victorious through the best way I knew how: prayer, guidance and a change in my perspective on life.

One way to do this was through "sitting on a couch" and sorting things out, otherwise known as therapy. I know many don't believe in it, but trust me it's not just for the "crazy" people. It works.

Yes, I had God and I'm a professional who has self diagnosed (thanks to WebMD) LOL. However, I realize that for the change in perspective I needed, a combination of the three would be PERFECT! You wouldn't believe how that changed many things. My life became full of twist and turns, upsets, peaks and now stable but FREE.

FREE from pain,
FREE from suffering,
FREE from self pity,
FREE to gain my life back,
FREE to be a warrior,
FREE to be available for greatness.

This approach helped me do some mental cleaning and allowed me to see my self-worth and act on the things that would help me be the best ME I can be. Perspective is everything!!!

THE COURAGE TO START AGAIN

As a victim of child sexual abuse, my self-worth was very low and the first place this manifested itself was the fuel and activity that I gave to my body. Naturally the first thing I decided to do was face one of my biggest challenges, working out and eating better. It was the best and worst thing that I could do at that time. It was the worst because I was afraid that I wouldn't keep up and fall deeper into self-pity. The best because to my surprise and fifty plus workouts later, with over seventy new Food Creations, I made it.

Then, in July 2011, I became pregnant with my second child. I lost the baby and had to deal with the pain and thought of not having something I've wanted. So what happened? I ate and fell back into the slump of not wanting to workout. I didn't care about much for the remaining part of the year. Needless to say I gained back the 20 pounds I had worked hard to lose in early 2011.

In January 2012, I found the courage to start again! I was not about to let obesity rule me or take my life. I began using my foundational principles from the nutrition boot camp and the important elements of working hard when working out. This time my Aunt and Momma were on the sidelines asking to get involved and I had to be an inspiration to them. I started going back to the gym and that was great but felt like I needed to face a fear of mine. That fear was a different type of activity, running. I have run for many different reasons (military, cross country in college) in my life and always HATED it because I was being forced to do it. I always finished last and it made me feel horrible. Then I was introduced to a running group called Black Girls Run (BGR)!

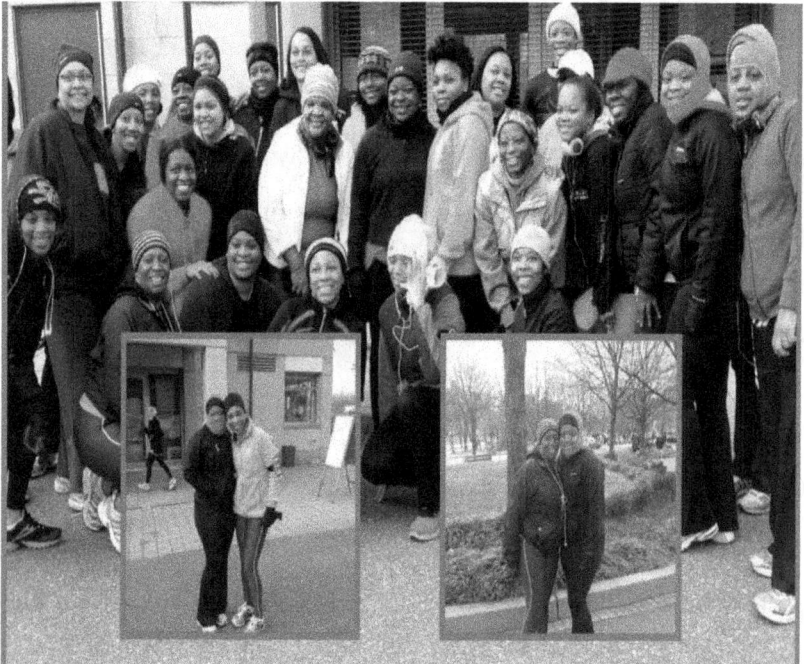

THE COURAGE TO START AGAIN

I began interacting with the group via FaceBook but not making the meet-ups because I was scared of my fear to run and the fact that I would be so slow. The great thing about getting started this time was, I wasn't alone. My Momma and my Auntie were trying to do it too. It was becoming a family affair.

Now today, 200 miles later, I may run slowly but I finish. Running has helped me mentally and has become therapy for me. BGR has been such a great support group as a supplement to my journey to becoming a better me. I have decreased my risk for Heart Disease by losing five inches off my waist, and losing 10 percent of my body weight. I am confident that this is no hoax, it's a permanent change that I truly enjoy. I am currently living a healthy, mentally, physically and spiritual life.

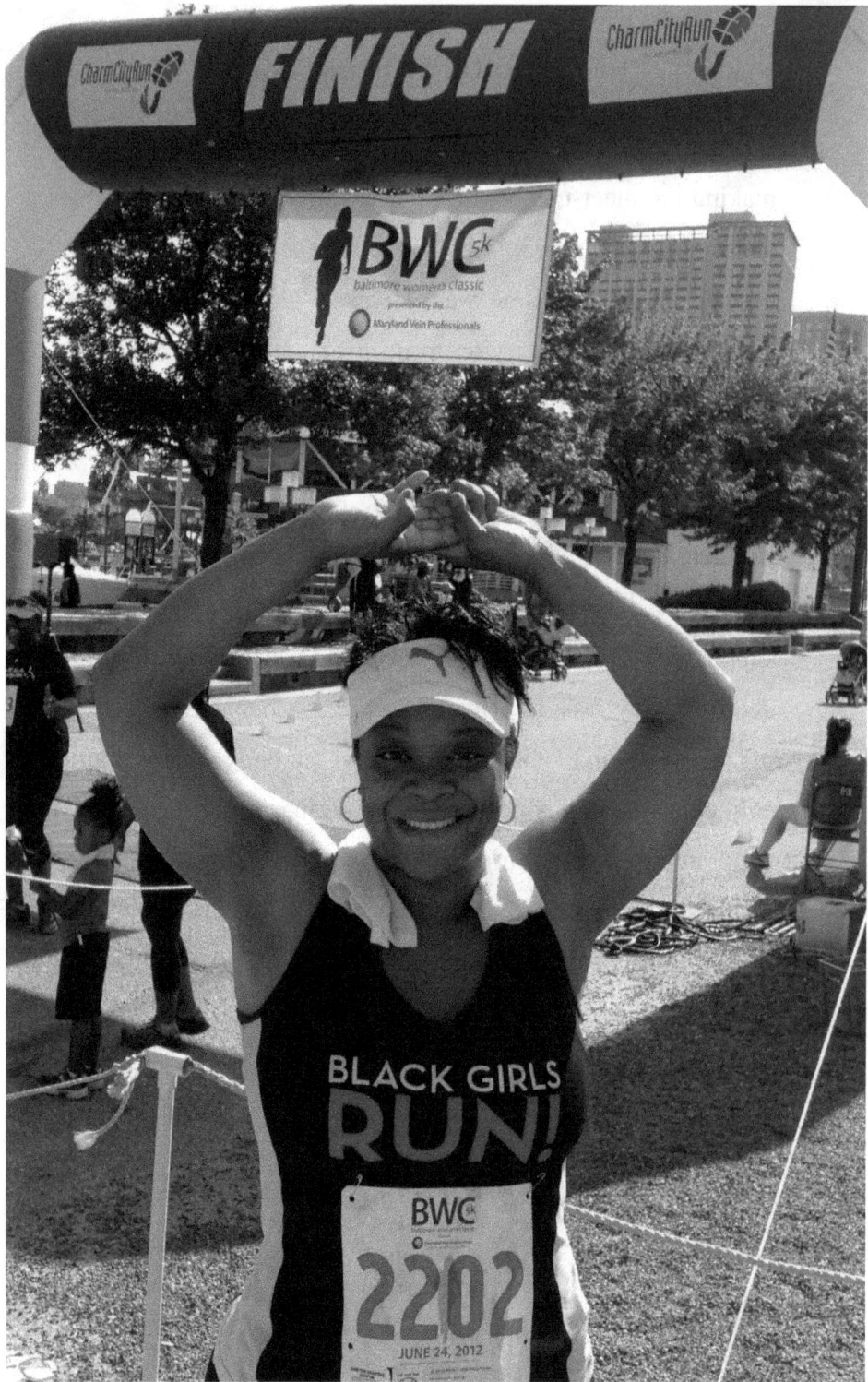

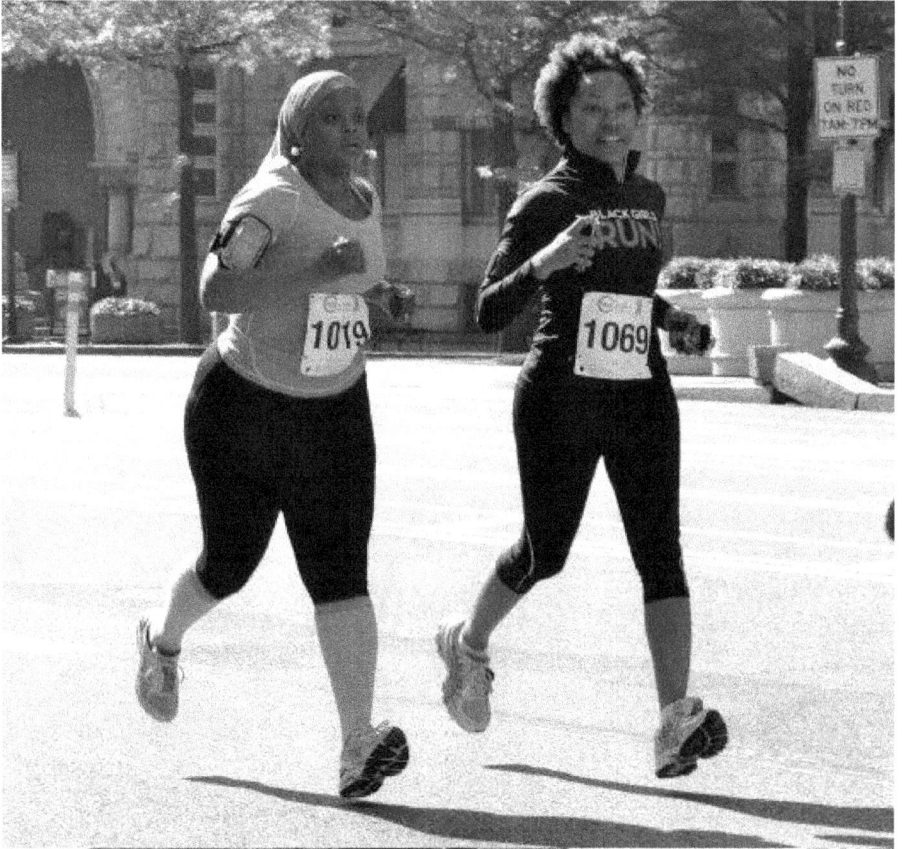
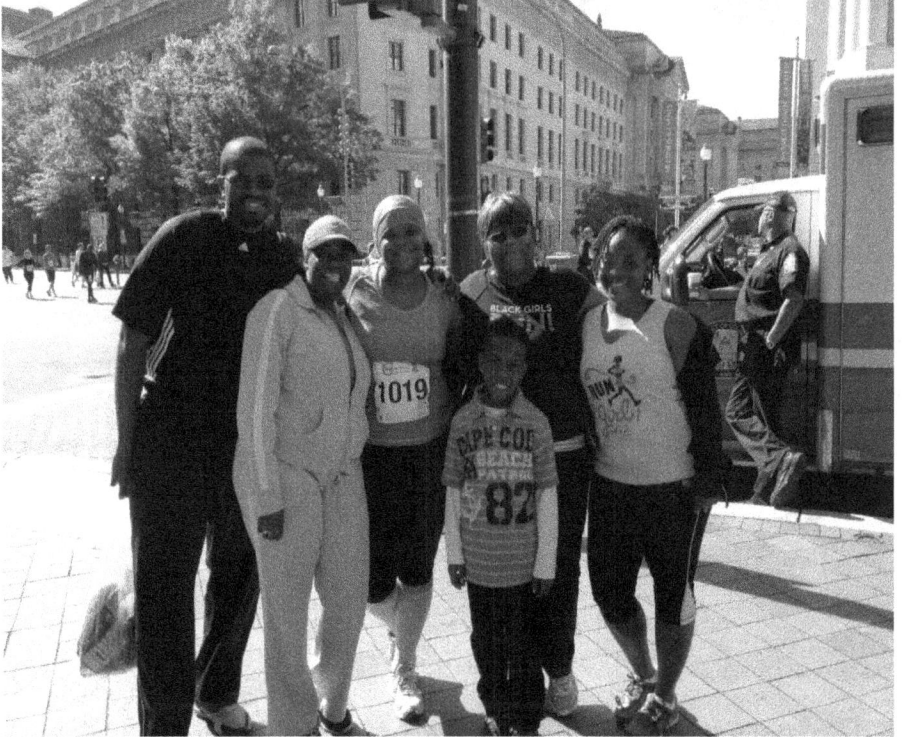

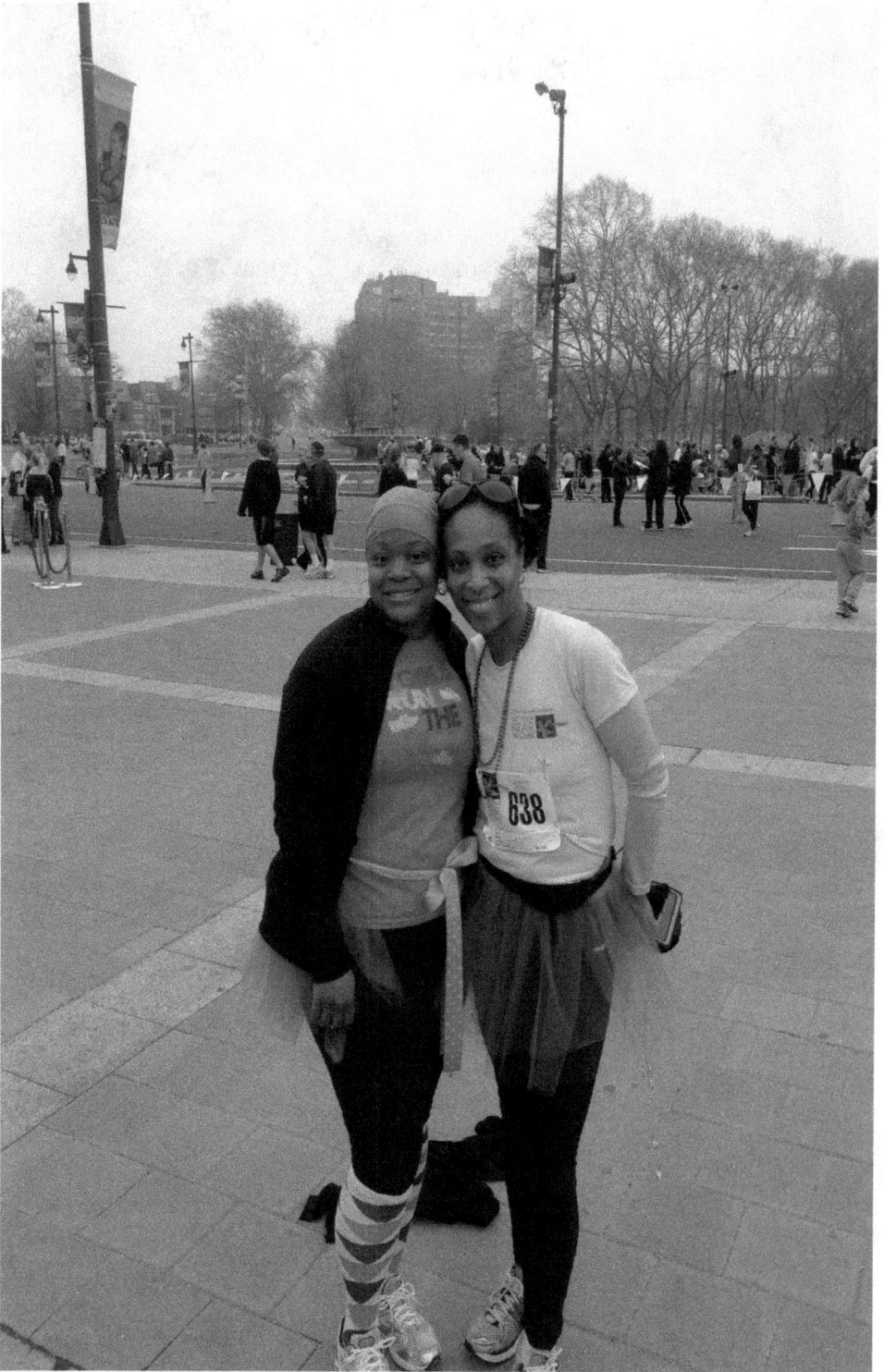

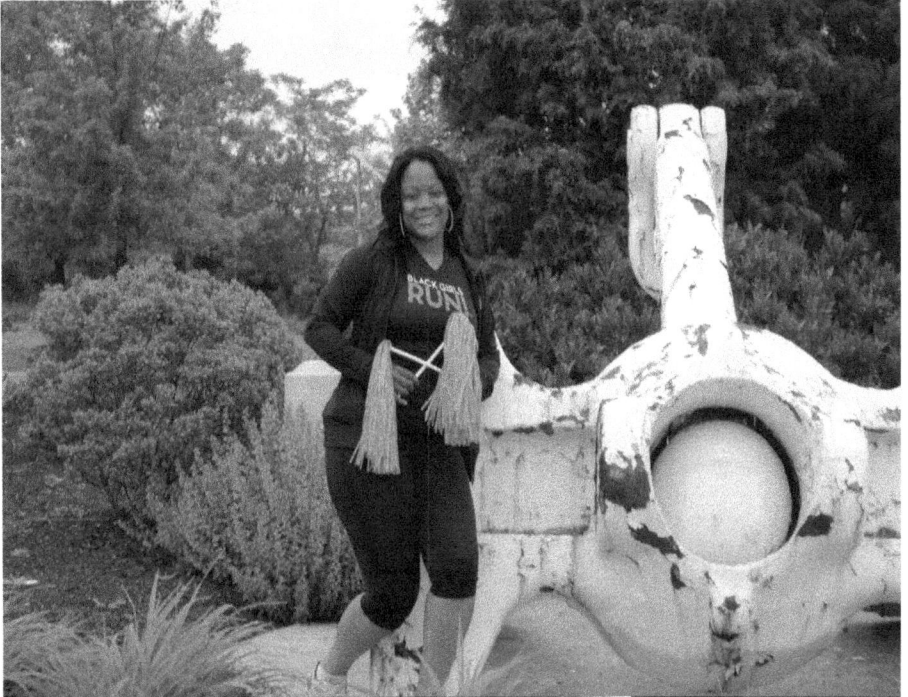
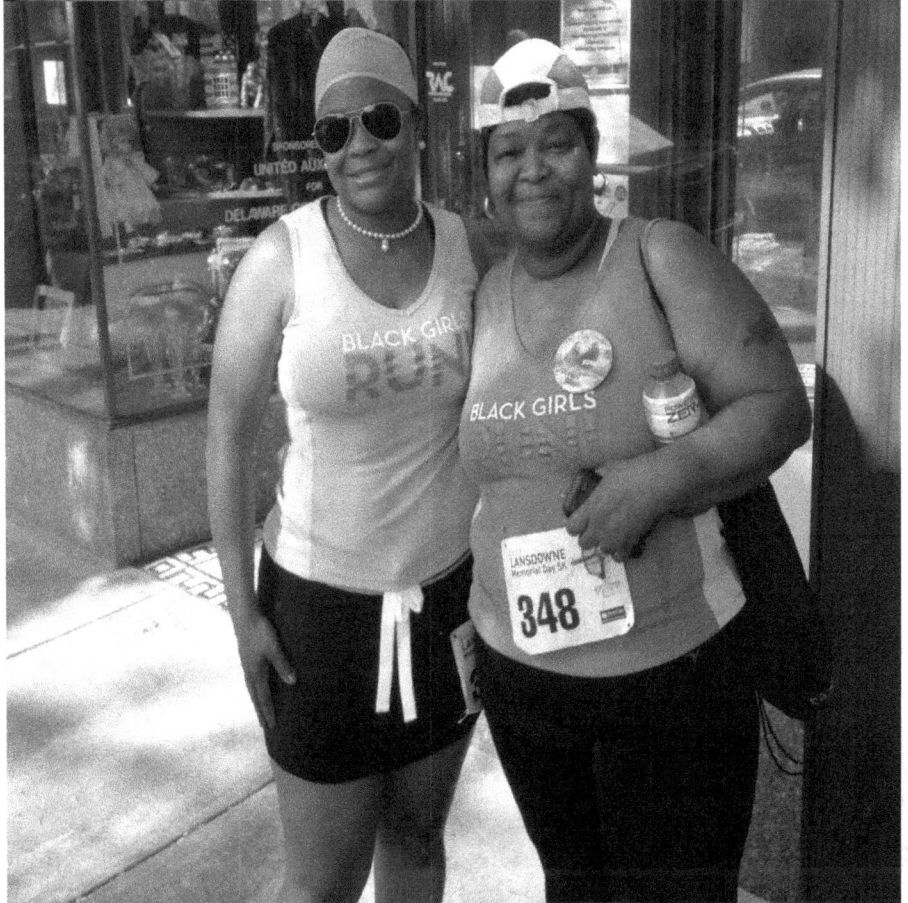

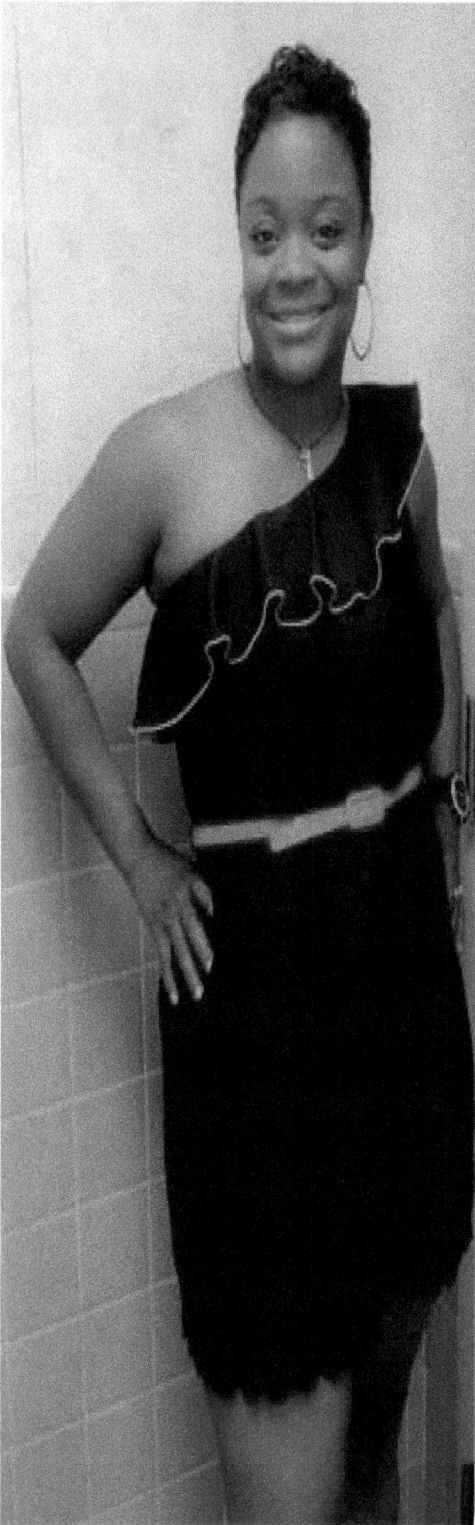

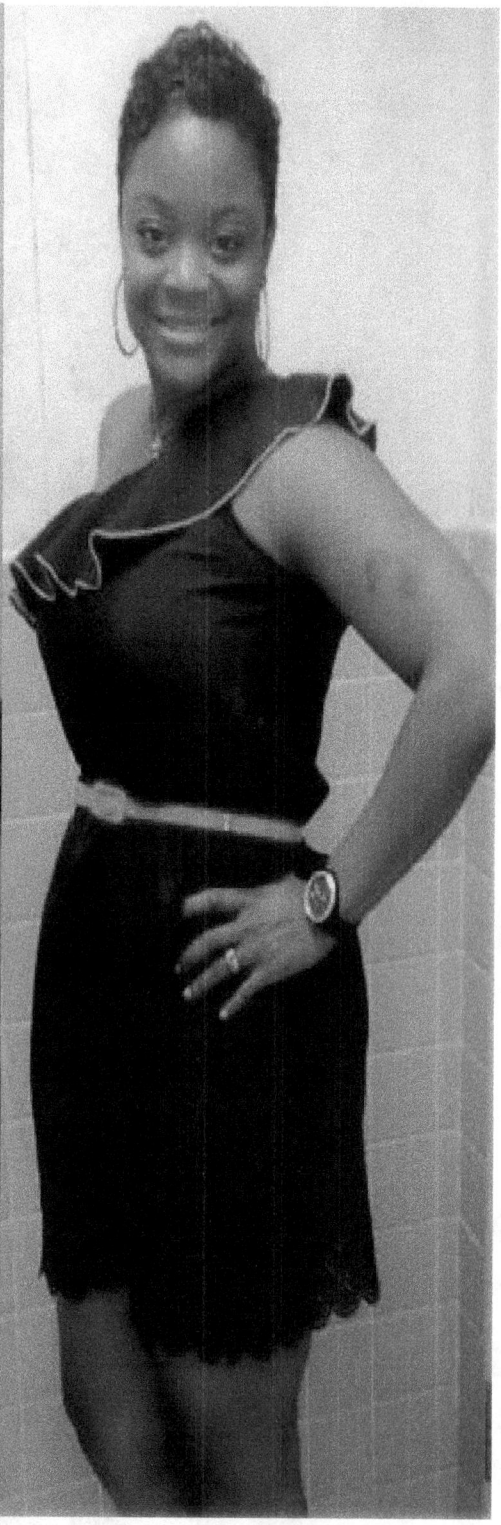

Nakia has been on a mission to reclaim her life through nutrition and fitness since December 2010. She started a Fan Page on Facebook, Food Creations by Nakia displaying many of her easy, simple dishes. She believes in a holistic approach to reversing the cycle of obesity in working from the inside out. Mental wellness is equally important as physical wellness. She enjoys running and cross training activities.

To date, she has completed five races this year in order to contribute physically and financially to a worthy cause. She has been a living testimony that slow and steady wins the race.

Education: She holds a BS in Rehabilitation Services, PSU (98') and a MS in Health Administration/Health Education, SJU (05')

THE "IT" FACTOR

FOREWORD

by MESSENGER ANNETTE M. CARSWELL

Many people want to do "it." Many people say they will do "it." However, "it" is often a mere image wedged deep in the hopes of many. Without the proper awareness of the necessary sacrifice, many are unable to complete the transformation needed to succeed. We all have been at a place where we felt disconnected from the proverbial "it" and watched as we then went spiraling into vicious cycles of disappointment. So when you find someone who did "it" and is able to share her miraculous journey with others, you jump at the chance to celebrate such an "It Woman!"

The message for everyone seeking to transform his or her bodies must first be completed in the mind. It is there where many of the decisions take place long before one gym item is purchased or barbell raised. It is in the mind where decisions are made for a better future and a better you. It is in the seat of control where you reckon with the last time "it" will detain you from your real you.

There you possess the needed fortitude and strength to belt out the last mile, or the chew on the not so pleasant carrots and celery. I learned this through our author and God's "It Girl" - Pastor Ramona Gaines. By observing her process from a distance, I watched her make some of the most serious alterations of her adult life. I saw the transformation long before it was noticeable in inches as she triumphed in her decision and choices to be all that God desired.

When "it" has dragged you through the channels of years of frustrations, fears, and failures and you finally become released from the battle of the mind, there is no way you can hold "it" or not share "it" with the world!

Please intake and exhale all this woman of God shares in this latest installment of conquering her "it." In doing so, you will feel inspired and driven to make a commitment to seize whatever "it" is that is seemingly trying to overtake your desire for transformation.

This is the journal many of you need to begin your process to your day of victory. This is your season of overcoming and possessing control over the "it" in your life. I implore you to become the next "It Girl" in your own life! Pastor Ramona did and is living proof for us all.

TIRED OF HIDING

I am WALKING in the newness of life.

I LOVE myself.

I CELEBRATE myself.

The grown mature woman in me

has learned how to comfort

and give the little girl in me

everything that she needs.

RAMONA M. GAINES

TIRED OF HIDING

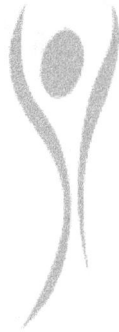

Yesterday, I cried for the little girl who was never able to be a little girl. As the tears streamed down my face and the sobs became uncontrollable, I heard the Holy Spirit say, "Reclaim and recapture what the canker worm, the palmerworm and the locust came to destroy." I thought to myself, "How can I go back?" The Holy Ghost then said, "I am restoring the years even now! Go get your life back now and Live!"

I wrote those thoughts on the morning of April 29, 2012 and ever since that day that is exactly what I have been doing. When I get up every morning, I embrace every day as a new day that has been given to me as a gift. That is not how it has always been, but I am choosing to be intentional about the pair of lenses that I view my life through. My name is Ramona M. Gaines and welcome to the story of my journey and how "Movement IS Medicine" has and is still influencing my life.

In June of 2011, I had to fly home to California for the Home going service of my uncle who had passed away. My flight was very comfortable because I ended up in a three-seat row all by myself, so I had plenty of room to stretch out and did not have to worry about me overlapping in anyone's seat. When I arrived in California I had no idea how my life was about to change, but it did in many ways. When I saw my family that I had not seen in many years, a few things became very evident. First, that they were very happy to see me, but I could also see the worry and concern on their faces because of my drastic weight gain.

Seeing them again brought back many painful memories. The last time I had seen many of them was when my

TIRED OF HIDING

Grandmother passed in 1995. Until the passing of my Uncle we had only limited contact, except for the Uncle who had just passed. He always kept up with me no matter where I was in life and I loved him for that.

While in California, every time we traveled somewhere in a car, no one would allow me to sit in the back seat. I thought to myself, "I know I can fit back there, why won't they let me?" Then I realized it was because of my weight and the size of the car. My feelings were hurt and I felt ashamed that I had allowed myself to gain so much weight. Then I kept hearing this still small voice say, "You are not honoring your body, you are not honoring your body." It made me sad and I cried a lot because I just did not know what to do. I did not know where to start at this point. I was also healing from a fractured ankle injury that I suffered at work. My mobility was limited at best. I made a promise to myself that when I got home I would begin to do something.

I cried out to God and I kept asking Him to not leave me like this. I kept begging Him, pleading with Him to help me. I knew then that I was getting tired of hiding and was ready to deal with the pain of my past. While in California, I asked my uncle, "Why did they leave us like they did when my Grandmother died? Why didn't we hear from them anymore?" His reply was, "You all were alright you had your mother". I responded, "No we didn't, and it has been hard and very lonely." I knew then that I was dealing once again with abandonment issues and it was one of the contributing factors of my emotional and binge eating.

When I returned home, I went to see my psychologist. I told her about my time with my family and the things that I had discovered about the women in my family lineage, or as some call it, pathology. Pathology is like your DNA. It is something that is unknowingly passed down from generation to generation. During my trip to California, I discovered many things that I thought I was alone in, were passed down to me. Some of those things included; low self-esteem, low self-worth and value, and loving one's self. I began to understand that loving one's self would change how you not only treated yourself, but also how you allow others to treat you. It also would change what foods you put in your mouth when you knew what the outcome would be. It would change the people you allow in your life and personal space. It would change whether or not you demand respect or just let people continue the cycle of mishandling you in abusive ways, whether they are emotional, mental or spiritual.

As we began to delve more into this new information, I was challenged to begin to break many cycles if I wanted a different ending to the story. It was important not only for myself, but for my daughter also. I began to wonder from my daughter's perspective what it was like to live with a mother who suffered with severe anxiety and mild depression.

These are the trauma lenses that I viewed life through;

1) Trust no one because they will let you down.
2) I was afraid of healthy relationships with men
because of the trauma I encountered after
being raped and molested by two different MALES.

During this time I met my third physical therapist and told him all my ailments due to my ankle injury. I love Jerry because he treated my whole body not just physically but he also heard and addressed my concerns about my weight. He was very instrumental in helping me create a new eating plan to remake my life. I began to implement his recommendations: a half of grapefruit before every meal, more fruits and fresh vegetables more water and get proper rest. Rest is so important for the body because it gives your metabolism time to reset. I also had to continue to regurgitate all the mess I had swallowed and allowed to fester on the inside of me.

My Psychologist was very instrumental for me in this season of my life. In my first session with her she asked me a question that made me want to punch her out! She asked, "How long have you been this big?" I looked at her with such anger and rage! How dare she say that! Thinking back on it, what a disservice she would have done me had she not. She was the only one in my life that was willing to address the elephant in the room.

Once I realized she was not backing down from that question I replied, "For about 12 or 13 years at that point."

She then asked, "What happened back at that time in your life?"

With tears in my eyes, I replied, "My grandmother died."

She then asked me another question, "Are you mad at her for dying?"

I replied, "Yes".

"Why?" she asked.

"Because she was the only person in my life that I knew without a shadow of a doubt that loved me unconditionally," I answered.

Her next statement as she reached for a box of tissues was, "You are still grieving."

I tearfully sobbed, "Yes."

I cried that day like a newborn baby as if it was happening all over again. The weight isolated me from people, yet it comforted me all at the same time. I was walking through life holding my breath and not living, just purely existing.

From that day forward, we began an excavation (digging up), of many deep hidden things that I was holding on to and had not allowed any light to hit for many years, going all the way back to my early childhood. It was as if I was waking up from a deep slumber and my senses were now alive. I could see differently, I was hearing differently and even my sensations were heightened by this coming alive experience. It was almost as if I was being reborn. In actuality, it is exactly what was happening. God was showing me that He was not going to leave me in the state that I was in. He was giving me beauty for my ashes, and I had many ashes to come through.

In February of 2012, I went to the gym to sign for my membership. When they asked for the initial payment, I went to reach for my wallet and my daughter stopped me stating, "I got this Mom." Talk about tears coming to my eyes and being proud of who she was! It was in that moment that I knew I had to do this. This gesture told me that my baby wanted me around. She wanted her Mom to live and be healthy. I went full throttle from that day and haven't stopped yet. At this point, since July 2011, I had already lost 46 pounds and did not know it until I went to the doctors. My doctor was elated. So much so, she slowly began weaning me off my blood pressure medicine by cutting the dosage in half. I was so excited, I was finally seeing progress. God was doing what He said He would do.

There is a saying that says, "When the student is ready the teacher shows up." I had to acknowledge all the other times I was just not ready. I was not ready to confront the pain of my past. I was not ready to confront my fears. I was not ready to say out loud I was mad at my Grandmother for leaving me. I was not ready to call myself on my behaviors that were detrimental to my well being. I kept entering into new relationships with different people with the same dysfunctional patterns. I began to tell myself to "shut up" when I heard thoughts in my head that were contrary to what the Word of God said about me. It's okay to sometimes tell yourself to just, "Shut-Up" and mean it. I also had to say to myself, "If you love yourself, then you will not stay up late and eat things that you know are not good for you when you are stressed, lonely or feeling depressed. You will stop self-medicating and deal with the issues that are confronting you in your life. You will show-up and be present because this is your life it is a gift that God has given you and you will not throw it back up in His face as if to say it is not good enough and you do not want it anymore." That is what I was doing every time I wallowed in self-pity, despair and entertained thoughts of suicide.

In March of 2012, I saw a piece on the news about a running group called Black Girls Run. I was so inspired by the motto of the group "no woman left behind". The woman who was interviewed shared her story on how this group helped to save her life. I went to find them on face book and asked to become a member of the group. I did not immediately go out to meet them. I was initially worried about how my ankle would fair on the concrete, but knew I would walk with them one day. One morning, I got up and decided I was going to go down to the meet up and see what is was about. It was around five something in the morning and I was wondering around on Kelly Drive trying to find the location. The group had already left, so I started walking, hoping to find them. Unable to locate them, I began to walk back discouraged because I did not see anyone. In a matter of a few moments, someone appeared and asked me if I was looking for Black Girls Run. I said, "Yes, but I guess I missed them." She said, "Come on, I'll walk with you." The rest is history.

That was on March 27, 2012. I showed up at a Saturday meet-up, still self-conscious about my shorts riding up in the middle. I remember one of the women saying to me, "Don't worry about what you look like, just keep moving." As I moved along, someone else would say, "Good job!" Someone else would say, "I am proud of you!" and it just went on and on. At the end of my walk, I was overwhelmed and in tears, this was too much. Where in the world did these people come from? They were so inspiring and so encouraging. I believed that I could do it, I really did.

I kept coming out.

I kept walking and many times I wanted to quit. I wanted to give-up. This was just too hard, I would say to God. One morning He replied with great force, "Where are you going if you quit?" "Who are you going to blame then, because it will be you quitting on you!" He then said, "Haven't I always been here? Haven't I always taken care of you and carried you?" At this point I was sweating and crying and it had all mixed together. He then told me to put on an old song that I had on my iPod and keep it moving. The song, "Can't Look Back Now" by Rev. Milton Brunson, was one that I had listened to many times over the years during my darkest days. The chorus says, "Carried me safely, never leave me lonely." I put it on repeat and kept on going to the end of my workout. When I was finishing up my wog (combination of walking and jogging) I saw my BGR sisters at the end, waiting and cheering for me. I stayed in my zone because I was hanging onto the words of the song for dear life.

He was speaking to me. Telling me He was still going to carry me safely and never leave me lonely. Although I had thought and believed I had been alone all this time, I knew now, I was not. God has always been there through all of my ups and downs. At that time I was only able to do two miles. I am now able to do three miles. I have lost 87 pounds and inches and am 13 pounds shy of reaching my first goal of 100 pounds. My highest weight was 323 pounds and I am 4 '11 ½ inches tall. That was a recipe for a Heart Attack, Stroke and diabetes. I am a walking miracle that was designed and created by God. He is the architect of this journey that I am on to wellness. Who I am is not defined by what I have been through, not the molestation, not the rape, not being teased by peers, not being a single unwed mother or anything. It is what God says that I am that matters and I am learning to embrace every day.

I am walking in the newness of life. I love myself. I celebrate myself. The grown mature woman in me has learned how to comfort and give the little girl in me everything that she needs. I don't have to be fearful or afraid of anything because God, my Father is the architect of my journey.

MOVEMENT IS MEDICINE

Movement IS my Medicine, the psychologist wanted to put me on medication to help me cope with my life. However, I cried out to God in prayer. He has given me all the medicine I need, and it is through movement. When your body starts moving and exercising, it releases the endorphins needed to relax your mind, help you cope and deal with stress. I no longer have to run to food. I can now make different choices and keep it moving. If you do not believe it, try it. Put one foot in front of the other and begin to move something and watch God take it from there.

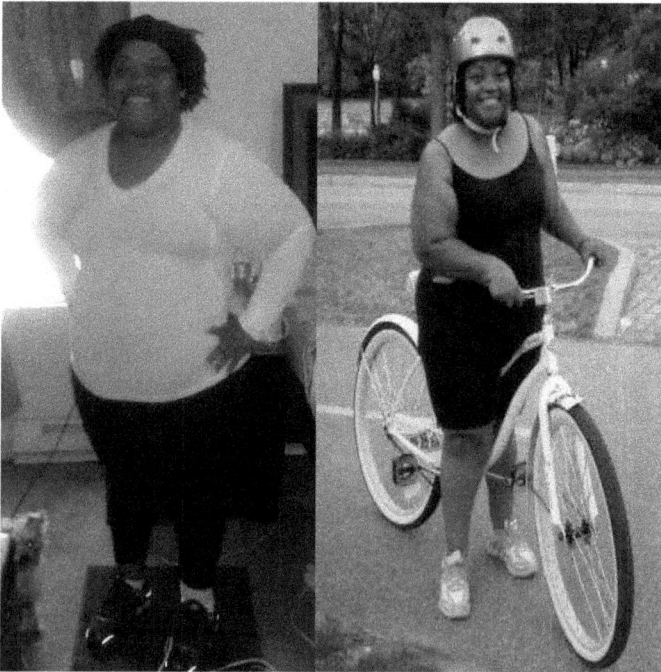

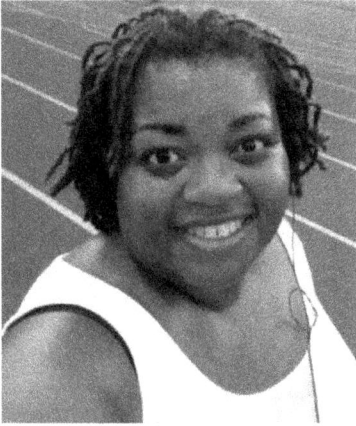

Ramona is the mother of a beautiful daughter, Ellana Monae Gaines. The eldest of her mother's three children and has a host of nieces and nephews.

Ramona M. Gaines, who is the Visionary for Movement IS Medicine, was born in Philadelphia, Pennsylvania. Ramona attended St. Ignatius of Loyola grade school, and graduated from Cecilian Academy High School for Girls. Ramona continued her education at Millersville University with her major being Radio and Television Broadcasting. Ramona also studied Biblical Studies at Manna Bible Institute. In 1999, she was Licensed and Ordained as a Pastor. She is currently under the leadership of Apostle Otis L. and Messenger Annette M. Carswell of Potters House Ministries of Pittsburgh, Pa. She has travelled for ministry extensively throughout the United States as well as Europe and Africa.

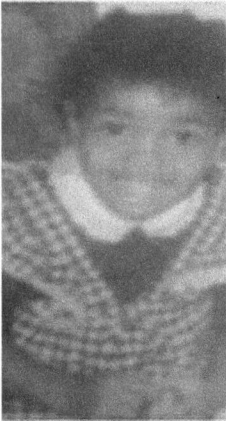

Ramona holds her certification as a trained Trauma Specialist with the Institute of Family Professionals through Lakeside Education Network.

Ramona is the founder and CEO of Styllwater's Café Inc. and Styllwater's Ministries. This ministry is a non-profit organization that provides a venue for Christian artists to share their gifts, connect with other artists and fellowship. Ramona is also the author of *The Styllwaters Story,* which details the accounts of her life leading up to the conception of Styllwaters Café.

Ramona M. Gaines is gainfully employed as a Parent Education Consultant for her own company, Parent Kids Network. God is using her to restore and transform the lives of parents and children, by imparting family structures and values back into the community.

Connect with Ramona:
prgaines23@gmail.com
styllwaters23@yahoo.com
www.styllwaters.com

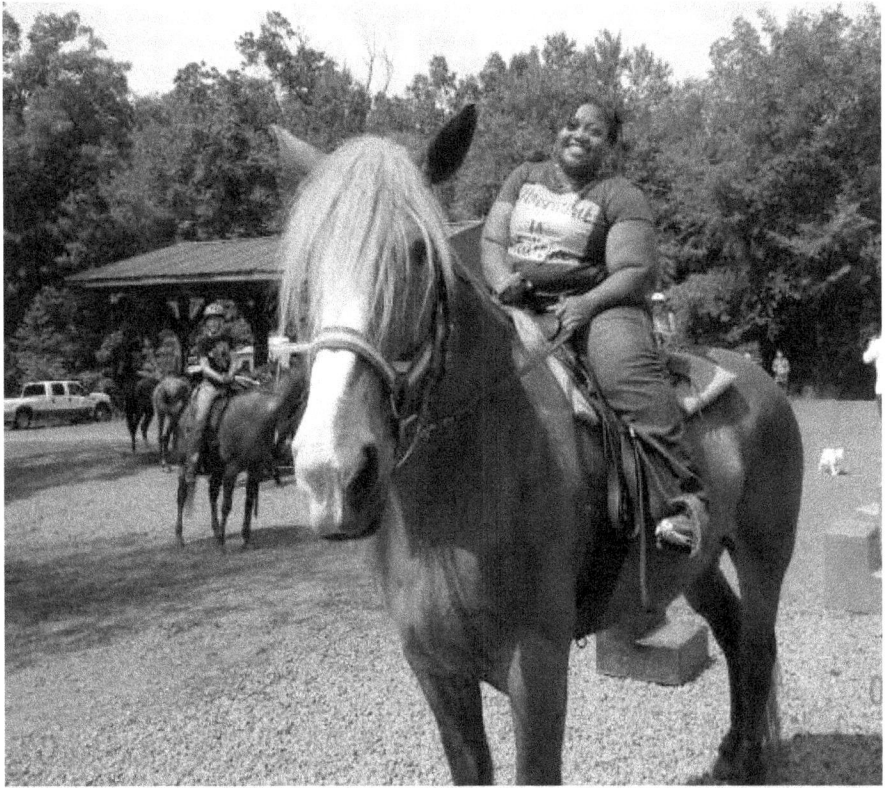

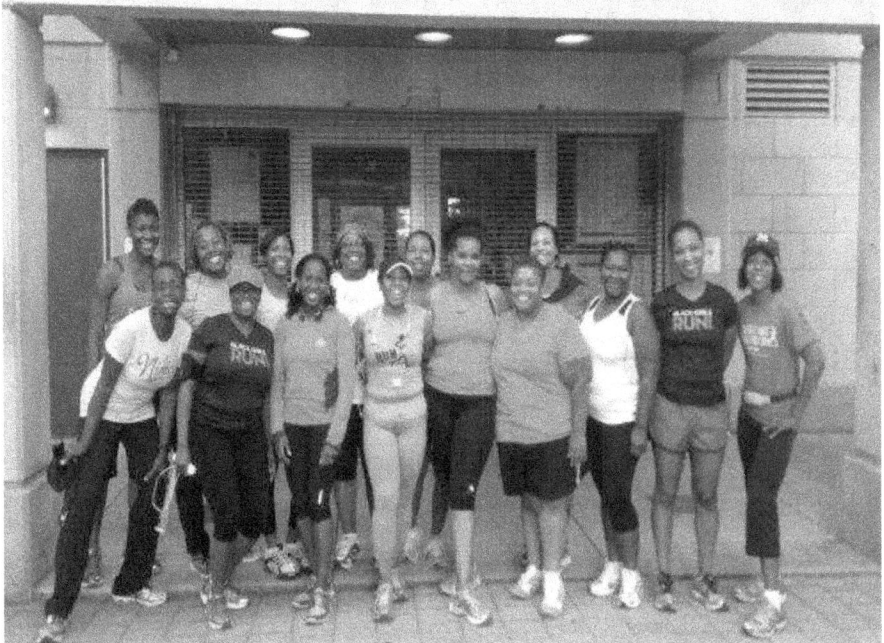

LLOYD HALL

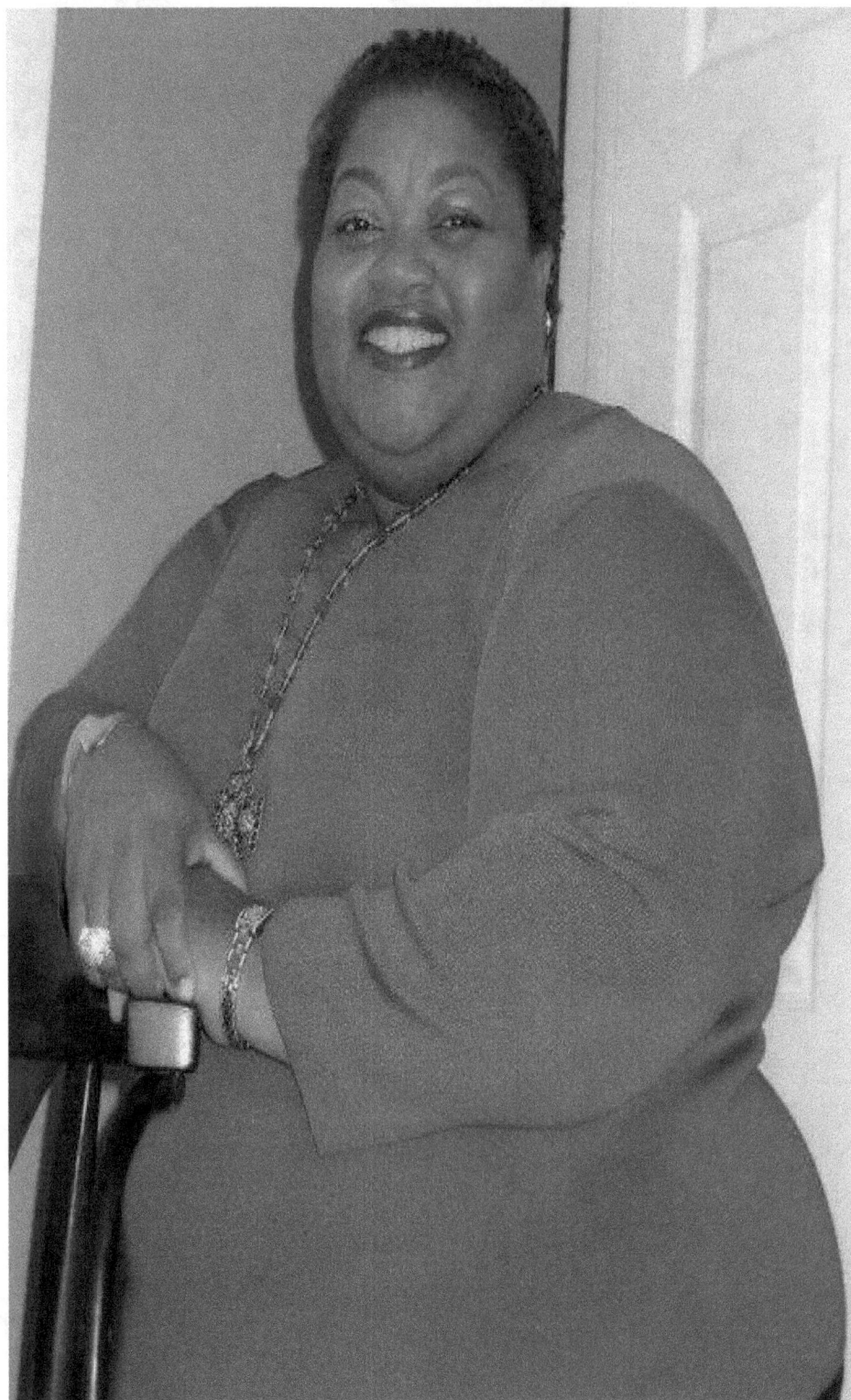

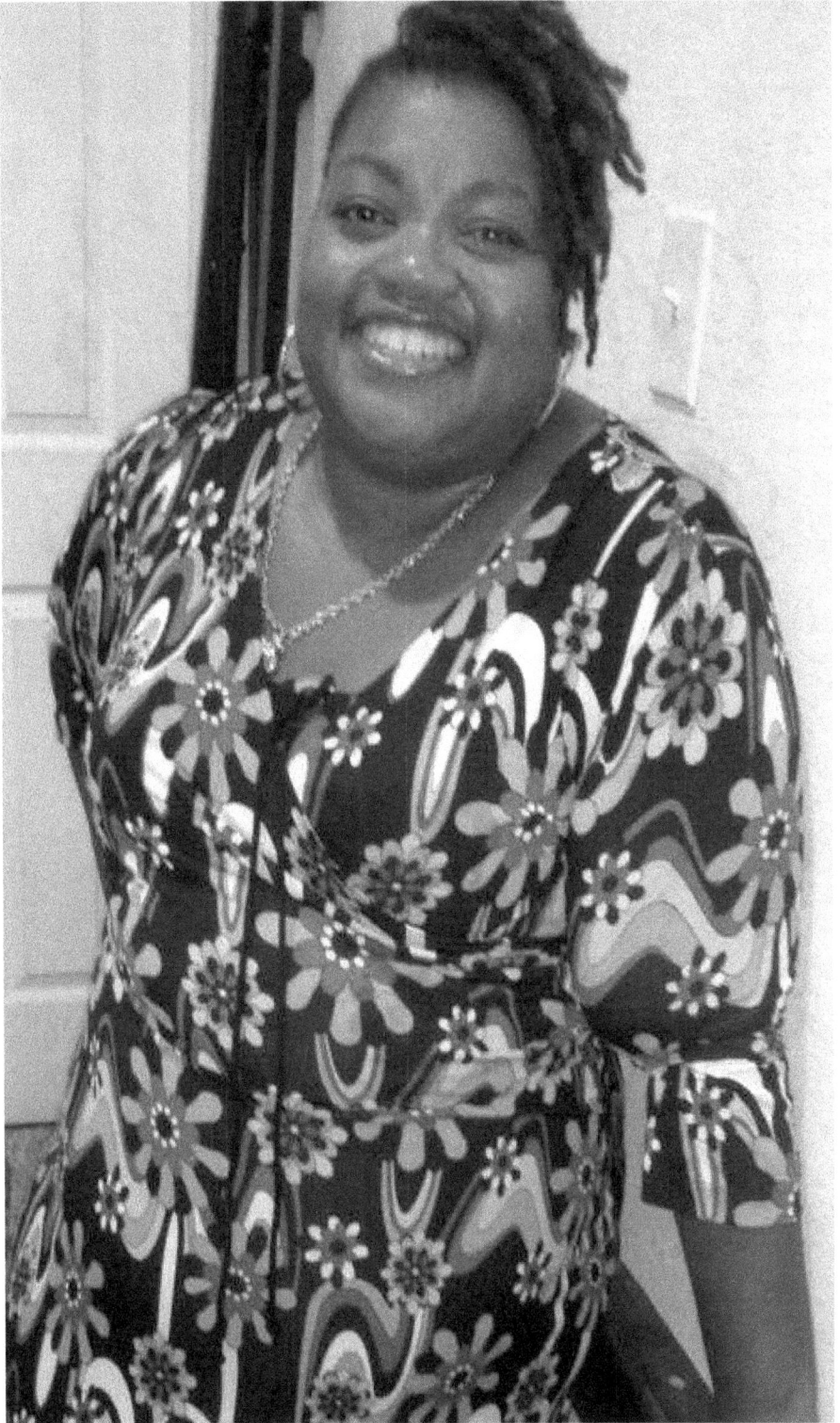

Ramona's Reflections

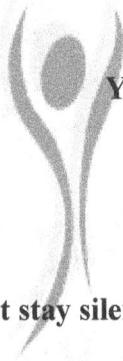

You've turned my mourning
into dancing again
and lifted my sorrows.

I can't stay silent, I MUST sing, for His Joy has COME!

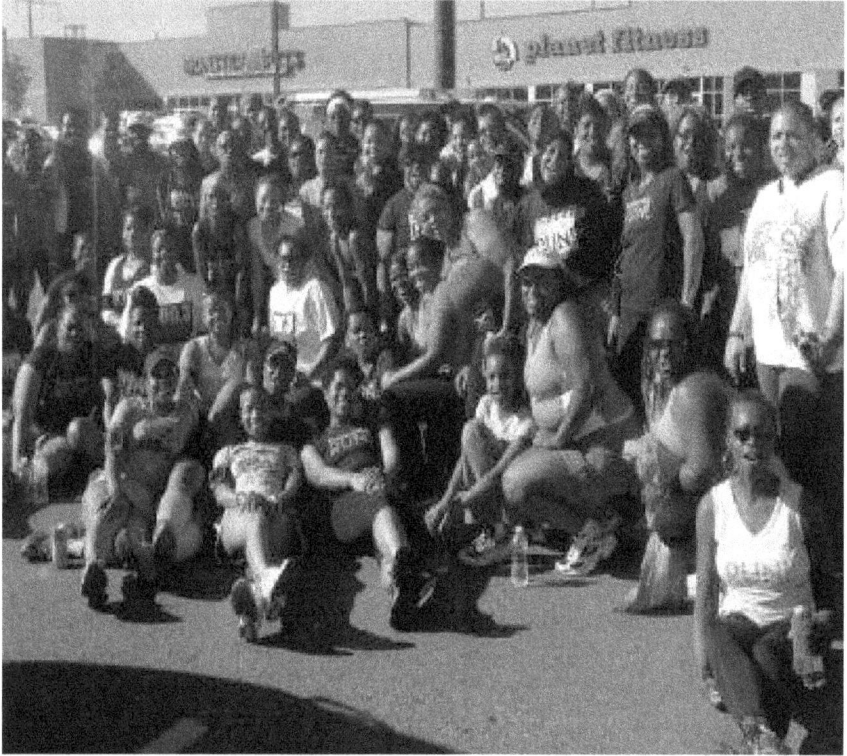

I officially joined the 3 mile club today. Participated in the BGR Hood run today and was able to wog (walk and jog) 3.2 miles this morning. Loving the God that I serve He keeps on doing GREAT things for me! As I ran by Church's Chicken I yelled out, "You can have your fat back!" That felt so good. Yes I am crazy but this is my story, this is my journey......have a great day family!

Lessons in "womaning up" are never ending. I am forever learning and growing each and every day. When the student is ready the teacher does show up. #momentofgratitude

We all start with an "in the beginning", which we have no control over. Then there is the middle or what some like to refer to as a "climax." I choose to still consider it the middle. Why? It is at that point that I cannot go back and rewrite the beginning, but I can take the pen and begin to write my own ending. By writing my own future, I mean taking responsibility for my own thoughts, decisions and actions, which will determine my outcome. Destiny does not just happen, it comes from a life lived with purpose, not perfection, but purposed.

People sometimes have a strange way of telling you they admire your strength, courage and determination. It sometimes comes out in their bitter drips of sarcasm or that needling poking thing they do to see if they can get a rise out of you. Thank you for letting me know indirectly you admire my courage and chutzpa (style), but I get it from my Daddy, who is the Giver of all good gifts. He is no respecter of persons so if you ask Him, He can do the same for you too! My name is Ramona M. Gaines and I approve of this message.com.

RAMONA'S *REFLECTIONS*

Lessons I am learning these days:
Life does get better,
but you have to hold on and keep pressing.

Hard work and perseverance does pay off.

Discipline is something you just cannot get through life
without having and putting into practice.

God REALLY is a rewarder
to those who diligently seek HIM.

God will give you beauty for your ashes.

YOU can be born again!

When you are the 'Dreamer', many will try to kill you. For if they kill you, they believe that the dream then dies. However, there is life even in death. Whatever the forms of death that have been in your life, always keep in mind the power of Christ; the resurrected One, still resides on the inside of you and has the power to raise the dream and the Dreamer from the dead.

MOVEMENT IS MEDICINE

When God is changing the set in your life don't fight it, embrace it. He knows what props you no longer need in your life and what cast of characters need to be killed off.

I do not want my living to be in vain. My Grandmom Henrietta always told me to just help somebody, and that is all I ever want to do. That is why when I find or experience something that I know will bless somebody, I am going to shout it from the mountain top. Jesus and Black Girls Run is what I am going to keep yelling so our women can save their lives and fulfill their God-given purpose in the Earth. Thy Kingdom come, thy will be done on Earth as it is in Heaven. His will is done through us because God uses us as agents of change to usher His Kingdom into the Earth.

I am finally home. I had a very full day today. Thanking God for travelling mercies and for entering into unchartered territories and realms of the Spirit today. When you are able to ascend in a corporate setting and begin to pull down the blessings of the Lord for God's people it is an awesome thing. Today in the Spirit I saw God literally loosening people and setting them free to go forth in Him. Destiny awaits you people of God, no matter how long it may seem to take you to get there. Delayed still does not mean denied. It only means God wants to ensure that you will be able to hold, contain and sustain what He is about to release to you. Are YOU ready?

When you grow up not knowing who you are,
not believing you will go far...
It leaves you feeling broken in the midst of your dreams
always chasing after the next moving stream
only to find it does not always dump into the next river or
even make it to the widest ocean
when you wish you just had a token
so you could get onto the next door open of a bus
because you believe in the next city it must be so much
better than looking at this old
raggedy dust that just keeps recycling itself
in the recesses of my mind as I try and try

to find a piece of the world that I can call all mine.... ....

MOVEMENT IS MEDICINE

Many of the times that I was discouraged, I said it was because I did not have anyone to help or guide me. My truth is, I just was not ready....Selah~

Good morning family, so glad to see another day. Getting ready to hit that pavement on the Drive with my BGR family. Still a little sore, but we're gonna make it do what it do and leave all the results up to God. Have an awesome day and most importantly remember, Movement IS Medicine!

You know, I always say, "What can separate me from my morning wog (walking and jogging)?" Today a skunk almost did. He was sitting in the middle of the Drive in the direction I would have to be going. I started running back and was like "shut the front door!" He eventually went back in the bushes. Other people went running by, so I thought it was safe and kept on going. It made me think of late night Tundra runs at the Ville. The skunks would be out thick sometimes, snicker snicker :)

You carried me safely, never leave me lonely. Oh, you carried me in the cradle of your arms. Oh in the midnight hours, when the tears are streaming down, when my friends walked out on me. In spite of what the devil meant for my harm, God meant it for my good.

This morning was a hard press, but by the grace of God I was able to do it. Weight is hard to pick up and move. I was about to stop in the middle, quit and cry. On the inside, I was telling God, this is too hard. Then I heard an old song come up from out of my spirit man, "I'm a soldier in the army of the Lord, I'm a soldier in the army". So I picked up my pace while I sang, thought about a soldiers cadence and was able to make it through. Then I saw my sisters from BGR swarm in on me like a host of angels and helped me run it in to the finish line and finish strong.

Alright, alright, alright! Getting this train moving this morning on my way to the Drive to meet my BGR sisters and then back home for breakfast and on to worship.

MOVEMENT IS MEDICINE

In everything give thanks for this is the will of God in Christ Jesus concerning you.

You've come too far from where you were to go back. Let God bless you real GOOD and keep it moving!!!

So I am in a very reflective mode today as you can see from my posts so I have decided to continue to let it flow. As I was sitting here listening to my Wedding song, no I am not married yet but I have picked out several songs already. Don't act like some of you have not done this too :) Any who, it is on repeat and I am listening to the words. Many of the words in the song are in the vows the bride and groom recite to each other. As I am listening, wondering can one really make these promises this thought comes to mind; How many have made these vows to another person and yet have not made the same vow to themselves. Have you vowed to cherish yourself in sickness and health, for better or worse, for richer or poor, til death do you part? If you cannot commit to you, how can you commit to someone else, if you don't take care of you? How can I believe you will care for me? We need to see the evidence of this before we make any lifetime commitments. You need to also be honest with yourself and say I am not ready if you have not first been committed to you. Honoring you begins with honoring the one who created you, God and following the instructions He has given you so that you may be in good health and prosper as your soul prospers. This is what establishes the balance and harmony many seek in others that should be coming from within instead outside of us. Many of us are divorced from ourselves already and then we invite another person into that broken union, expecting them to make it all better. This may be one of the reasons divorce is so easy to do for some. No one can complete you but Christ. A marriage is the union of to wholes not halves and it is God who does the meshing together, only then can the two become ONE.

Growing up I believed that love was forever. When you found that special someone, you fell in love, got married had children and it would be forever. As I grew up and experienced life, 'forever' seemed to evade me and slip through my fingers many times. As I was driving home yesterday, one of the songs that contributed to my "forever syndrome" came on the radio and I began to sing it as I once did in a childlike innocence. Then the woman in me spoke to the child in me and said, "Nothing is forever, things don't stay the same and neither do people, even with the best of intentions. The only thing I can guarantee you Ramona, is Jesus is the same, yesterday, today and forevermore. Love does not always make it to forever. Sometimes it stops, shifts or changes. His love is the only constant and consistent love you will have in this life. Now Ramona, I am sorry no one ever took the time to explain this to you, but today I choose to enlighten you, help to heal you and equip you with all the necessary tools to pursue, have and enjoy your abundant life with all of its ups and downs."

I just woke up from a dream about a TastyKake Lemon pie that had whipped cream icing on it. At first I just tried to eat a little bit of the icing until I got around to the center of the pie and realized it was my favorite, lemon!!! Man I better just get up and run. I'm running from the pie! I'm running from the pie! I'm running from the pie! I'm running from the pie! If anybody asks you what's the matter with me, just tell them I'm a recovering emotional eater and I'm running from the pie!

Not everyone is going to be happy for you, celebrate you, or support you. So get your noisemakers, throw your own party, and keep it moving!

Total weight loss to date since July, 46 pounds!!! I am so happy!!! Woohooo!!!

Okay family just wanted to keep you updated on my weight loss journey, I lost another 11 pounds. So the grand total now since July 2011 is 57 pounds down!!!! Doing the happy dance over here, come on and samba with me!

April 30- I had a pace partner on the Drive this morning and boy did she challenge me. In my mind I was like, God this is so hard. Then to finish up running it in I thought I would die. But I keep repeating to myself, "I can do all things through Christ that strengthens me, over and over again until I crossed the finish line. It is an awesome feeling to push past yourself and beyond your normal comfort zone.

May 30- My Big Bruh always reminds me that "Movement is Medicine" and that is true. However, movement is not always physical. In my journey of weight loss it not just about physical exercise but also the mental, spiritual and emotional exercise that is taking place. I began the inner work long before I saw any outer signs. I had emotional, mental, and spiritual "weight" to deal with. I had to begin to call myself on the carpet about a lot of things that were hindering me, the "inner me", and not the enemy. My "inner", was and sometimes is my biggest enemy. Forward movement takes work, but the results bring discipline and determination. Don't despise your journey, learn to embrace it and love it.

May 11-I just want to send a shout out to all my bones, muscles, and joints. Well my body period for showing up this morning and putting in the work so we can have a more perfect union. It is an awesome feeling when all cylinders are able to operate at optimum peak. I really appreciate you. To my God given mind, you are the bomb! You continue to give me the will, drive and desire to continue on and do what is best.

P.S. I think my left knee is mad at me, lol...

Come on sweetie I love you and I need you to survive!!!

May 14- Okay I think my body is on auto-pilot now. I clearly was ready to sleep in and go to the gym later instead of the Drive. The alarm went off, "Go Get It" by Mary Mary was playing and I got up and walked straight to the bathroom. Uhmmm, body thought we were tired but guess not! So let's go get it! Good morning people!

May 16- Two mile wog completed. Thanking God for one more day. Embracing my process even more and enjoying the journey. Have a great day today on purpose everyone!

May 23- The cheese curls in my glove compartment are calling my name! If I can just make it home to get to my veggies, I will be fine. Pray my strength family I only have about 8 blocks to go......

May 24- 2.0 miles done on the Drive shout out to my pace partner who pushed me to kick it up a notch. Interesting thing, she was humming a familiar song while we were walking, "That's When You Blessed Me". I thought to myself, Yes Lord! You are doing in my life just what you said you would do! So grateful and thankful for all these blessings! Peace and blessings to you all family. Remember, Movement is Medicine!

May 26- Thought of an old James Cleveland tune today, "I Don't Feel No Ways Tired, I've come to far from where I started from. Nobody told me the road would be easy. I know He did not bring me this far to leave me." I took a moment and looked back from where I was and where I am now, and my God you have been faithful, oh so faithful! Thank you Lord for ALL you've done for me!

May 25- Weight loss update: Drum roll please! For the month of April I loss 8 pounds, and for the month of May I lost 7 pounds! All totaled, that is 15 more down and 33 to my first goal weight. Let's get it!!!

March 31- Today while walking I made a decision to make a commitment to myself, for wholeness, healing and good health. I have done this for so many other people and things, but today, I said "Ramona commit to being the best YOU you can be! Cheer yourself on, motivate yourself and most of all, LOVE yourself!"

Man I am so proud of myself 2miles on the Drive this morning. God you are so awesome! You speak a word and it is so! Lord you said you would not leave me like this, but that you would perfect those things concerning me. You are a keeper of your word.

March 27- Did my first walk/jog with Black Girls Run this morning and it was awesome. Had a great sister beside me who helped me finish strong!

"That was a grueling workout, 35 minutes on treadmill and 30 minutes on step machine. I caught myself rolling my eyes at the step machine when I saw my inclines getting higher instead of lower. I so apologize, I know it is for my good baby, but it was not feeling good at the time. I promise I will do better tomorrow."

My Black Girls Run t-shirt is an xl! Last July I was wearing a 4X. Can you say happy, elated, encouraged and hopeful about my future!!!

"Did not make my early morning wog, off to the gym I go. The love affair continues we are beyond infatuation at this point. I have truly decided to give my all in this relationship. It is the only way I know to get the results I desire...."

Me and BB (Beautiful Butterfly, my bike) made it down to the Parkway and back all in one piece. I am exhausted and ready for bed!

Made it to the Drive this morning got my 3.1 miles in. Saw an old co-worker while jogging. I kept talking and by the time I realized it, I was finishing up, so I just ran it on in. She and her dog ran with me. That one snuck up on me but it was pretty cool to know I could. Have a great day everyone!

April 1-
Yesterday I did 2 miles, today I pushed the envelope and did 3 miles. When I got to the 1.5 mark, I was ready to call a cab a friend or somebody! Nevertheless, I pushed through and I made it! To God be the glory!

"Had and awesome wog on Kelly Drive this morning. Shout out to Francis for her first morning wog with BGR. I felt like I was channeling the spirit of Harriet Tubman this morning as we were wogging in the day break singing on the inside of me, "Us gon be free", and this is the way to freedom. This experience is so liberating! Thank you Lord!"

"I got my 2.5 miles in this morning on Kelly Drive. It was cold as jacks out there. I needed some gloves. How come when you get closer to finishing the benches in front of boathouses start looking like comfy couches? I just wanted to lay down. I began to see pillows that were not there :) Have a great day people and don't forget to get out and vote!"

STRONGER
THAN I THOUGHT

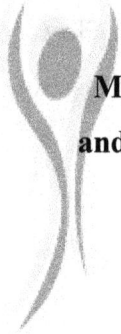

My journey has been one of great loss
and now I'm recovering my peace daily.

DEBI WILLIAMS

STRONGER
THAN I THOUGHT

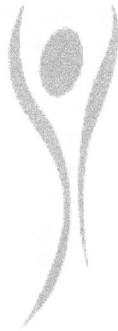

I have been walking since April to the present to work every day because I lost my car. Some might see this as being an inconvenience. However, not only did it promote weight loss, which I had been working at for sometime but it also gave me time with the Father. It is the best stress reliever for me and I have had the time I need to meditate and prepare for my day by the time I reach my destination.

To date I have lost 8 lbs. and learned that I am much stronger that I ever thought I was. My journey has been one of great loss and now I'm recovering my peace daily. Things truly don't matter, but being in the middle of God's will for my life is key. As believers, we should be holding on to His word for dear life because it is our lifeline

As I have gone through life, I tried to consult His Word, yet I have suffered. I lost my home of 10 years. I lost my automobile and I almost lost my will to fight. In these past 2 years I've experienced my Father in such a more excellent way. I will not die but live. As we move together, let us continue to make the Father proud one step at a time.

Be blessed & keep ***MOVING!!!***

Debi Williams

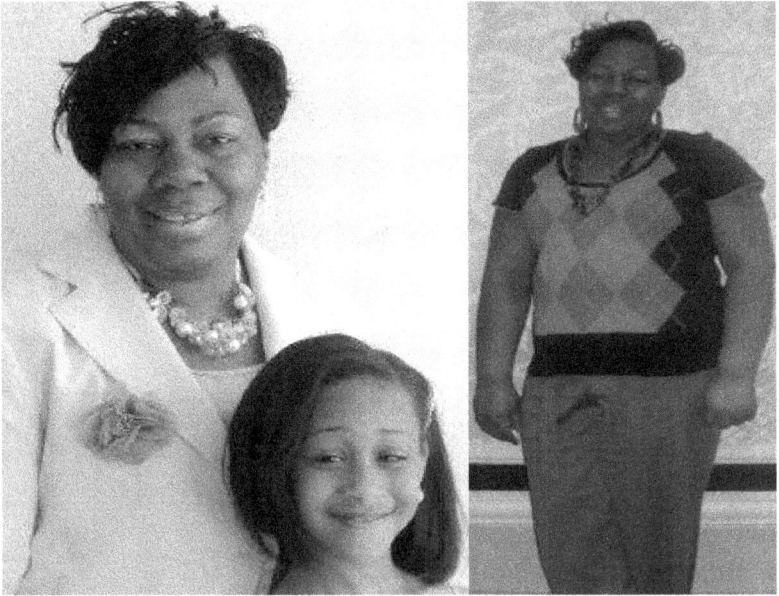

Debi Williams is an Educational Assistant at Samuel Smith School in Burlington, New Jersey. She earned her Bachelor of Arts Degree from Rutgers University. She loves to sing and encourage women of God. Her pastime is being an Event Planner.

BABY STEPS

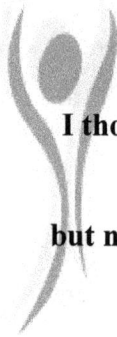

I wanted to cry for joy.
I thought I could start a healthy lifestyle
with a change of diet alone,
but now I know, it takes diet and exercise.

RENATA HUNTER

BABY STEPS

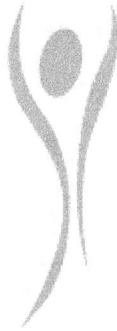

My movement began on June 22, 2009, when I lost my best friend and the father of my children as he was coming home from work on a Friday evening. The loss was tragic and devastating, however I learned to forgive, forget, and what it meant to be without the one that meant so much to making my family whole. I realized I needed to preserve my health and take my medical conditions more serious. It has been over 3 years, but the wounds from the lost are still there. Nevertheless, this is the beginning of my movement.

MOVEMENT IS MEDICINE

I was diagnosed with Diabetes and was in denial for many years. I often said, "How could I have this chronic disease and no one in my family has it?" My biggest challenge was food. I love food and I won't deny it. I was cautious of the food choices and tried to eat right. I did not pay too much attention to labels and went to numerous food and nutrition classes. After talking to a close friend who gave me so much encouragement, I realized I could do this. I suffered with the disease for years but did not want to accept the fact I really had it.

Within the last year I started going to a specialist. We discussed a new exercise plan, diet, and medication dosages. She suggested I should not make too big of a goal but start out with baby steps. Her encouragement led me to seek a personal trainer who encouraged me to take his supermarket shopping class at a local supermarket. As we walked through the aisles he showed me what to eat and why I should eat it. I picked what I ate and he did a comparison, showing why the product he selected was the one I should eat. It made sense. After the personal trainer became too expensive, I needed another form of exercise. I keep thinking of the encouragement my dear friend said to me and decided to join

Black Girls Run. The group is a group of inspirational, encouraging and motivational women with goals to promote a healthy lifestyle through movement.

Before it was time for my next doctor's visit, I received a message from my specialist stating, "We need you to come in the office." The call was alarming and I did not know what was wrong. I thought my blood sugar must be bad if she is calling me for an office visit. After two weeks passed, I finally decided to make the appointment to find out what was wrong. As I sat in the office patiently waiting, the doctor comes and we start having a casual conversation about my diet and exercise program. As she looked through my chart she said, "Well, I am so proud of you, you are right on track as we planned and your hemoglobin is coming down slowly. I see a big improvement, your pressure is good and you have lost some weight."

I wanted to cry for joy. Before that movement, I thought I could start a healthy lifestyle with a change of diet alone, but now I know it takes diet and exercise. The movement is the medicine I needed to kick start the change for improving my health and my life. "Movement IS Medicine."

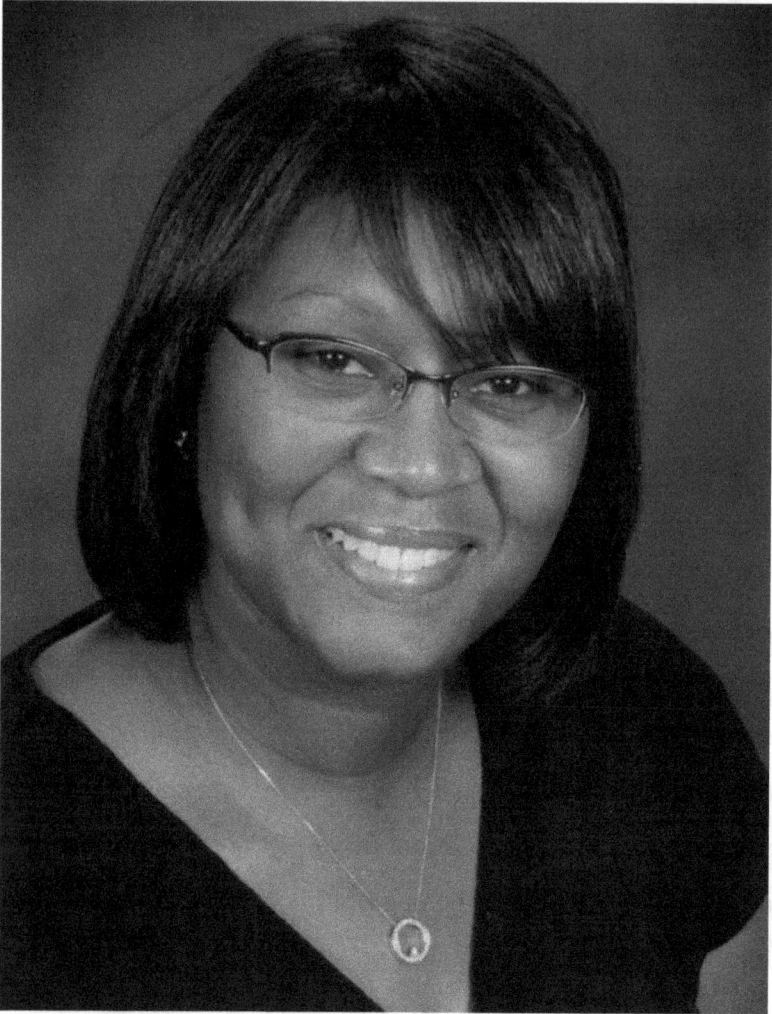

Renata Hunter is a native Philadelphian and a mother of two young men, 13 and 16years old. She is a full time Hospital Administrator and a part time student studying for a degree in Health Administration.

GET UP AND *MOVE* SOMETHING

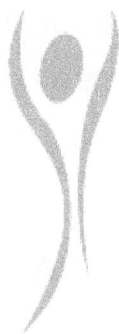

MY ENERGY

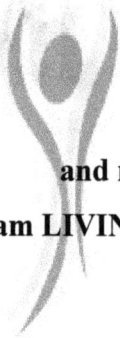

I FEEL better,

LOOK better

and my thoughts are with PURPOSE.

I am LIVING out my destiny of a healthy lifestyle.

EVON DELEE

MY ENERGY

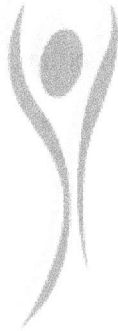

I started in January 2012 eating a clean diet, which consisted of fresh fruits and vegetables, baking all of my food or cooking in olive. I increased my water intake of maybe one glass a day to eight glasses a day.

I signed up for Planet Fitness Gym in February of 2012 and began to exercise. My starting weight was 262 lbs. and I now weigh 225 lbs. It was imperative that I began to work on my health because I had been diagnosed with hypertension and stress and was in poor health.

MOVEMENT IS MEDICINE

One of the most noticeable things that I experienced after this lifestyle change was that I now had energy. In March of 2012 my husband of 31 years began to also work out with me, so it is now a family affair.

This journey of wellness and holiest health of mind body and spirit has been very rewarding. *I feel better, look better and my thoughts are with purpose. I am living out my destiny of a healthy lifestyle.*

Blessings,
Pastor Evon Delee

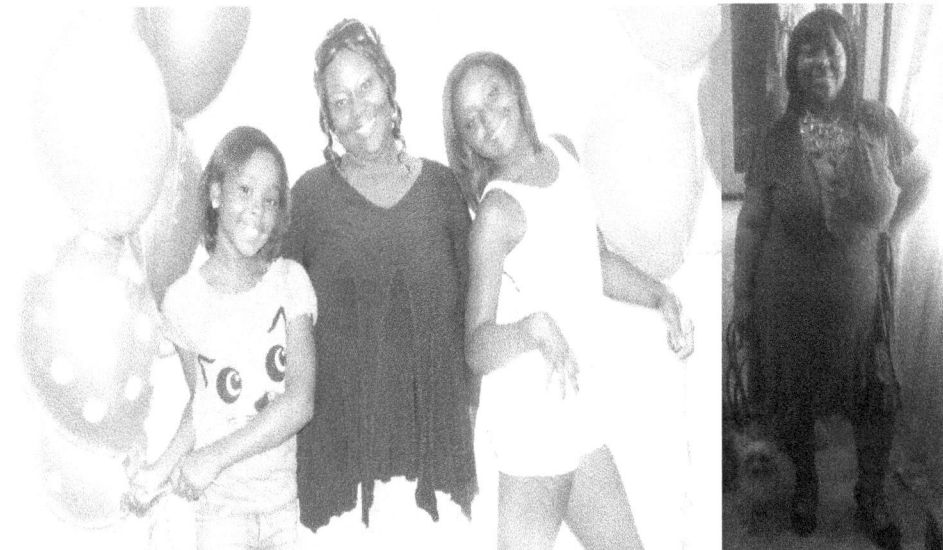
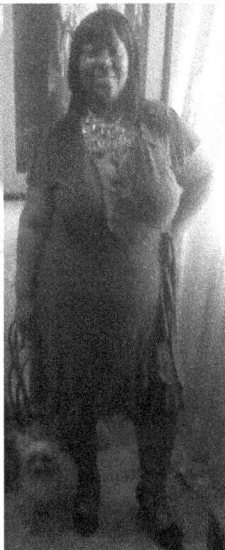
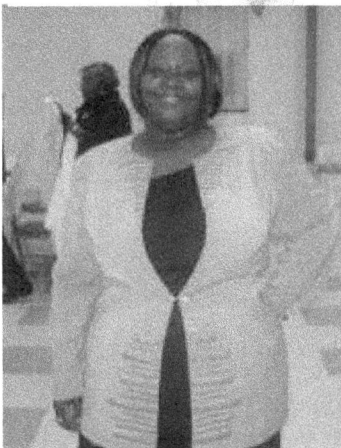
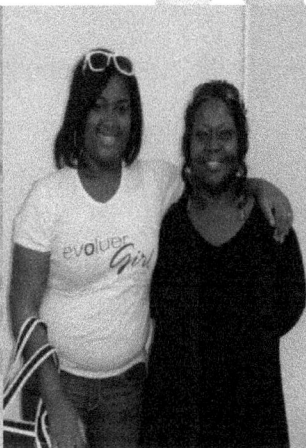
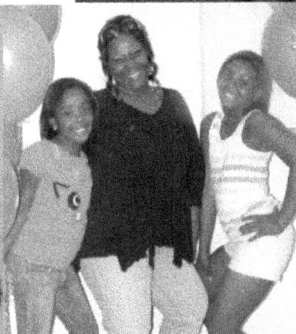
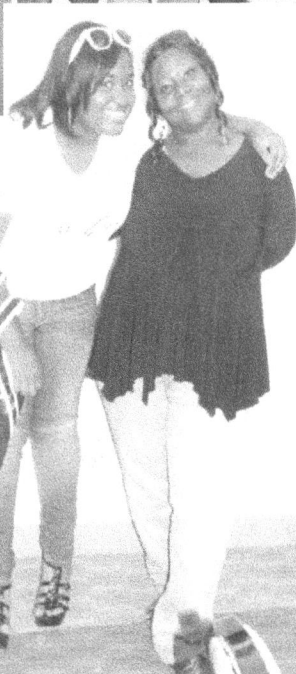
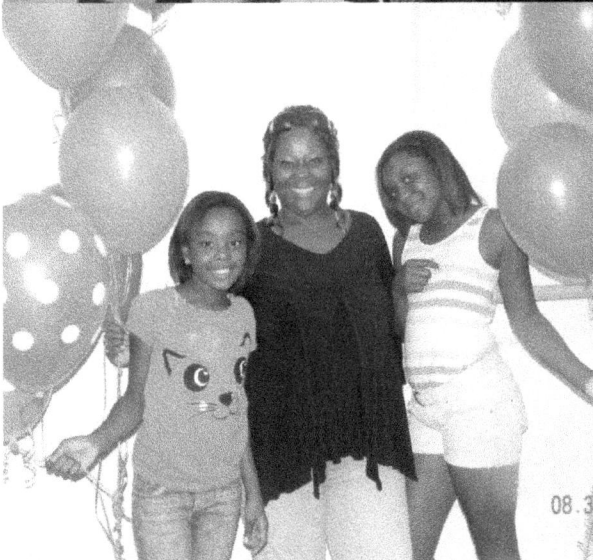

08.3

Pastor Evon Delee is the wife of her childhood sweetheart and husband of 31 years Glen Delee Sr., mother of two sons and six grandchildren whom she is very devoted to and loves to spend quality time with often.

In 2009 Evon retired from Glaxsco Smith Klein after working there for 25 years to work in full time ministry.

She is the assistant Pastor of The Church Down the Way, Program Director of Daughters Beautiful which serves at risk girls in the Mill Creek Community. Pastor Delee is committed to teaching and empowering young women about their inner beauty as well as their outer beauty and how to *"love the skin that you are in"!* Pastor Evon Delee is the National Evangelist for Potter's House Ministries Alliance under the leadership of the Apostle Otis L. and Messenger Annette M. Carswell of Pittsburgh, Pa, a Board Member of the Mill Creek Community Partnership and also serves on the Advisory Board of the Mill Creek Playground in Philadelphia, Pa. She has traveled extensively through Africa and Nova Scotia Canada doing Missions work with families and also in the medical missions field.

GET UP
AND *MOVE*
SOMETHING

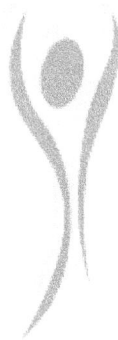

FINDING A BETTER ME

I did get to a great place of renewal and purpose!
I stand here today with a different mindset!
I am now ready to take on the world,
leave all of the baggage behind me
and start afresh!

ERIKA ALLEN LYNCH

FINDING A BETTER ME

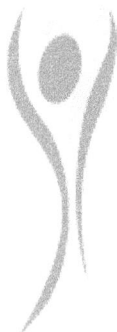

My story may differ from the other ladies in the book. There are so many emotions, with so little time to explain. I'll try my best. I am just starting another journey. I have only lost 11 pounds. I have been here several times before, however, this time I feel a little different. My journey is not just about the weight that I've carried all of my life. It is about finding the old me! Rather, finding a better me!! My quest will be for personal growth first and weight loss as well!

This journey will be to shed the pounds that weigh and slow me down, in addition to the other baggage that I carry that also weighs me down mentally, spiritually and physically!!! We have all been there!!

Thank you Jesus for the strength to move forward!! Jesus is my Doctor and Movement is Medicine!!! At the end of this journey, I will be a better, lighter me! In many ways, the BEST me that I can Be! A more focused me. A less stressed me. Back to an organized me. A less people pleaser me!! A focused, Christ Centered Me! A better Servant, Wife, Mother, Daughter, Sister, Aunt, Niece, Cousin, In-Law, Friend, Boss and employee! A better all around Me!! That's my goal!!! Am I there yet? No. Where do we go from here? I am a work in progress. After the hurt, after the pain, after betrayal, after 5 miscarriages, God has always kept me even through it all!

My story begins as an overweight happy child. I cannot tell you where it came from. I had an awesome, memorable childhood in West Oak Lane, Philadelphia! I would not change a thing! I cannot pinpoint or blame my weight on anything particular. I usually blame it on a few things. My mom was and still is a great cook! I had three older brothers and no sisters. I ate whatever my big brothers ate. I don't want to think of the portion sizes with that! Maybe one day I'll figure out what the true reason is or was, but for now, that's my story and I'm sticking to it!

It is also strange for me because although I was overweight, I never let it keep me from doing too much. I swam, roller-skated, loved to ride my bike, went to block parties, cheerleading and I always sang on choirs. Everything my friends did, I did too! I also had a cousin say to me that she thought my weight never bothered me because I would be the first one jumping in the pool! Although she was correct, what she didn't know was that I got in the pool quickly so no one would have time to stare! I was always mapping out plans. I was comfortable to a certain point with my weight, but I never liked being overweight. In junior high, my weight bothered me a little. Once in high school, it wasn't as bad because I had boyfriends or interests, so I wasn't an isolated overweight child. I was very confident on the outside, but always struggling a bit inside.

MOVEMENT IS MEDICINE

My first big quest with weight loss was when a male friend that I grew up with called me and said that his mother had shared with him that he should help me lose weight. As he talked with me, tears ran down my face. He never knew this part of the story. I was so embarrassed, but I was also grateful and appreciative that they thought that much of me to want to help me. Wiping my tears, my first weight loss quest began. We met early in the morning and walked from West Oak Lane to the Cedarbrook Mall, passed the Cheltenham Square mall and then returned back home! I have no idea how many miles we walked, but there is no way on God's Green earth I can imagine that walk today!

He was already thin, so when we arrived on Wadsworth Avenue, I would buy him donuts and I would get fruit for myself. We talked all the way there about our friends that we both liked at that time. He was a true a friend and I don't know if I ever told him how much that meant to me! I began exercising in my basement and I believe I went down almost 5 dress sizes. You couldn't tell me anything. I was super excited! All of the guys that I liked, who previously paid me no mind, were now interested. I thank God for keeping me focused!

I realize now that although I made progress, I did not make a lifestyle change. I later went back to my old ways of eating and eventually the weight came back. By College I was up a few sizes again. Like most, I continued on many quest to lose weight. Some were successful and some were a waste of time. I think one of the hard things for me, is that I always had such a good life; full of love, family and friends that my weight wasn't always on the forefront my mind. I was content with myself to a certain point. In College, I met the love of my life. My husband made me feel like the most beautiful person on earth. My weight wasn't really an issue. It would come to my mind from time to time, but I would try to forget it and continue with my crazy eating habits!

Twenty something years later, I found myself evaluating my life; the many ups and downs, the suffering of several miscarriages, the joys that God has blessed me with, my growth in the Lord and my family life. I am now a mother! Yes, God blessed us after 5 Miscarriages to have a beautiful daughter that reminds me that all things are possible if you place your faith and trust in HIM! Even in my happiness, I found myself in a dark place of depression, dealing or not dealing with some events that rocked my world over the years. I allowed them to be a stronghold over my life and just recently came to a place of renewal. *A TIME TO CONCENTRATE ON ME, SO I CAN BE A BETTER PERSON FOR ME AND EVERYONE ELSE!*

My husband went on a 2 week mission trip to Africa. This allowed me some quiet time to refocus, evaluate my life and think of an improvement plan. The two weeks went fast and I didn't get all of my accomplishments done. However, I did get to a great place of renewal and purpose! I stand here today with a different mindset! I am now ready to take on the world, leave all of the baggage behind me and start afresh on what God has in store for me and in store for my family!

I started exercising and changing some of my eating habits. It obviously was perfect timing. I began talking with Sister-friends on Facebook about our journey. So many of us where in the same place, trying to get in shape mentally and physically! Some were surpassing goals that I couldn't imagine and others, like myself, were just getting started. I have lost 11 pounds so far and although I am nowhere near where I need to be, I am on my way to a healthier and better me!

I will continue to persevere each day. I still find it hard to resist the weekend temptations, but I am sure after reading the other stories, you and I will be inspired to continue to MOVE because MOVEMENT IS MEDICINE!

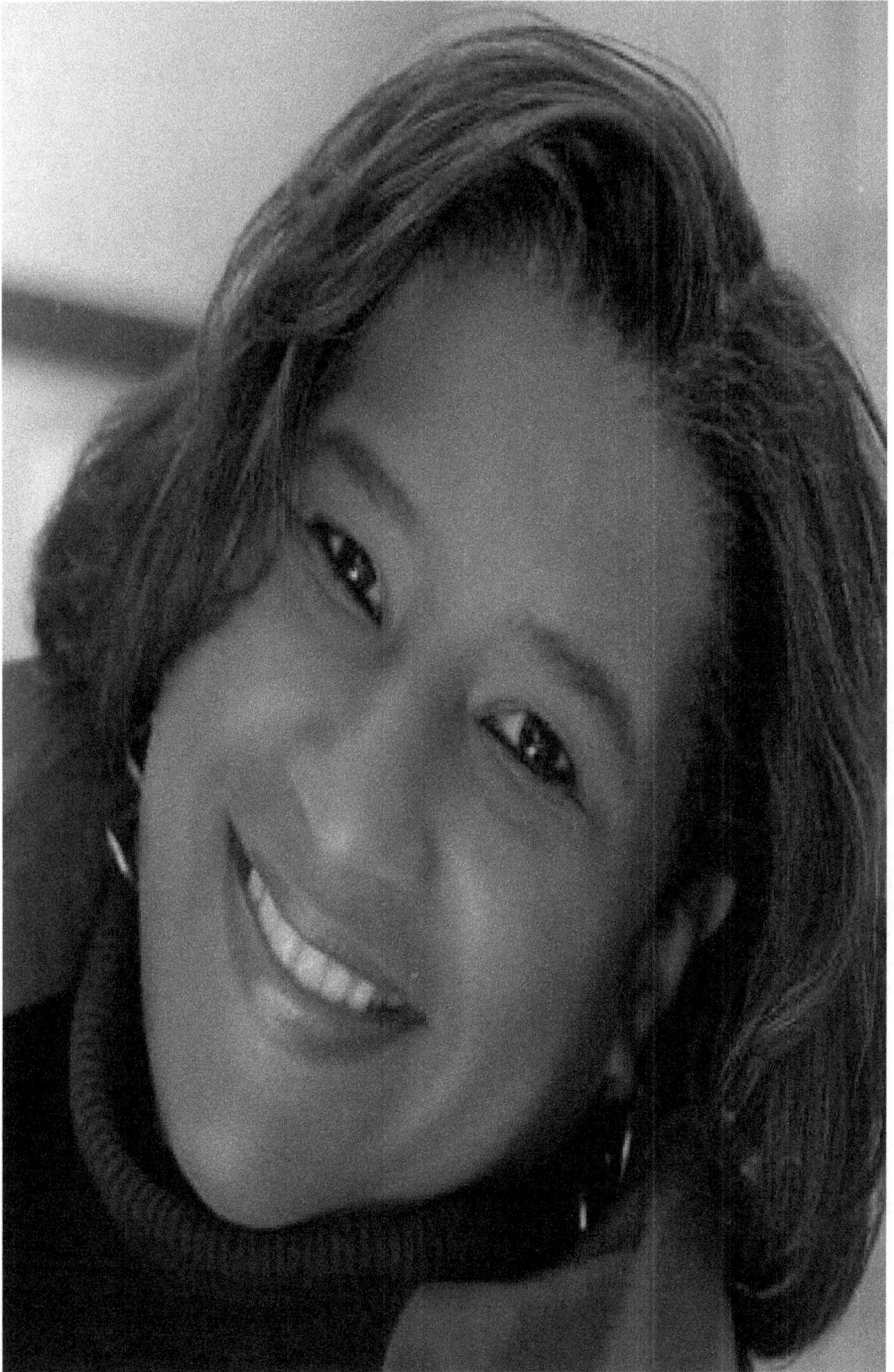

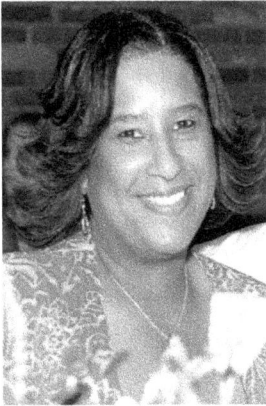

Erika Allen Lynch is a native of Philadelphia, PA and currently resides in the Coatesville area. She was educated in the Philadelphia Public School system. After graduating from Murrell Dobbins High School, she entered Millersville University and majored in Occupational Safety and Hygiene Management. While at Millersville, she became active in the Delta Sigma Theta Sorority, Millersville Gospel Choir, Omega Essence Club, Black Student Union, Minority Tour Guide and Black Greek Council.

After graduating from Millersville, she secured a position at Hahnemann University in Center City Philadelphia as the Safety Coordinator for the Hospital. In April of 1994 she was promoted to Regulatory Compliance Officer. In May of 1995, she became the Director of Health and Safety which involves ensuring that the Hospital and University is in compliance with the regulatory agencies that govern safety standards. Later that year, she was promoted to Director of Safety and Security and was responsible for environmental safety and security issues for the entire facility which is a 616 bed hospital with 12 buildings, over 5000 employees, 2000 students and 220 laboratories.

Mrs. Lynch is currently the Director of Environmental Health and Safety at Villanova University, which is a 225 acre campus, 80 buildings consisting of 10,000 students, and approximately 2500 faculty and staff.

Mrs. Lynch is a member of several professional organizations and in May of 2000 received her Master's Degree in Environmental Protection and Safety Management from Saint Joseph's University in Philadelphia.

Erika, her husband Joe and daughter Jordan are active members of Mt. Zion Baptist Church in Coatesville, PA under the leadership of Rev. H. Michael Boyd. She enjoys working with people, sharing the Gospel, and knows that there is so much work to be done. She looks forward to what God has in store for her and her family as they grow in the Lord.

Mrs. Lynch contributes her accomplishments to God above all, her parents and her husband Joe. Her favorite scripture is: Colossians 3:17 "AND WHATEVER YOU DO IN WORD OR DEED, DO ALL IN THE NAME OF THE LORD".

To God Be the Glory

for the Great things He does and will continue to do!!!

GET UP AND *MOVE* SOMETHING

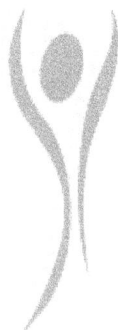

THE BIGGEST LOSER

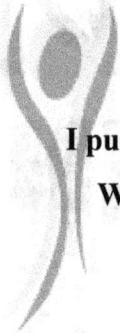

I put it in my mind that I was going to win.
Well, guess who won the competition?
I CAME IN FIRST PLACE!

SHEILA BYRD

THE BIGGEST LOSER

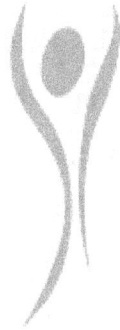

As far as I can remember I was a very skinny child growing up. I was called "BEAN POLE" because I was skinny and if the wind blew too hard I would blow down the street. I heard it all. My weight gain started after I was married and had two children. After I had gained weight, family and friends would say things like, "What happened to you? You need to lose weight, what size do you wear now?" It has been an uphill battle for me. I would do well for a while and then I would mess up. I'd lose some and then gain some. I'd lose some more and then I'd gain some more, so on and so on. I tried so many different diets, some worked and some didn't. After trying over and over I gave up and let it get the best of me.

By now my self esteem was shot. All I could hear was, "You are fat!" As I looked around, all of my friends and family were thin. I would go to the store and look at the clothes I used to wear hoping one day I would get back to that size. I tried to get back on track and change how I ate and what I ate. It worked for a while, and I did lose some weight. However, I lost focus and there I went, again, back where I started. Eating this and eating that, watching TV, eating late night snacks before I went to bed and not thinking about myself or my body. I got to the place where I didn't care. I justified weight by telling myself, "Fat is where it's at, no dog likes a bone."

For a long time I wouldn't do a thing, until my mother said to me very lovingly and nicely, "The more you put on, the harder it is to take it off." She had a weight problem as well. However, she had the means to go to a well known place to lose weight and kept it off until she passed away. A few years after the passing of my mom, I thought about what she said and I began to do something about my weight.

THE BIGGEST LOSER

While working at Medco, we had a BIGGEST LOSER competition and my team came in second place. I worked very hard on my weight and did very well. From that point on I did ok. My hairdresser also had a BIGGEST LOSER competition for cash prizes. I put it in my mind that I was going to win. Gym, LOOK OUT, HERE I COME! My sister and I would go at 7:00pm Monday thru Friday. Well, guess who won the competition? I came in first place! I lost 23 pounds and was able to wear some of my old clothes again!

I was so happy that I was able to lose that amount of weight. I wanted to keep on going. However, I started going backwards, doing the things I knew was wrong, but I just couldn't stop. The more I tried, the more I kept going downhill. Just as I was about to give up, my sister Carla called to see how I was doing with my weight loss. She attempted to encourage me by saying, "You can do it! I have faith in you!" At that moment I had to ask God to help me. Then, my other sister Ramona was on facebook talking about taking her life back and how she lost weight. I told myself, if she can do it, I can too!

MOVEMENT IS MEDICINE

I began to do what I could do indoors at home. My son
laughed at me for how I was exercising. I didn't care, I kept
on going. My sister Ramona put a fire under me as she got
smaller. It took me some time, but I got smaller also. I pray
this will help somebody.

DON'T GIVE UP!!!

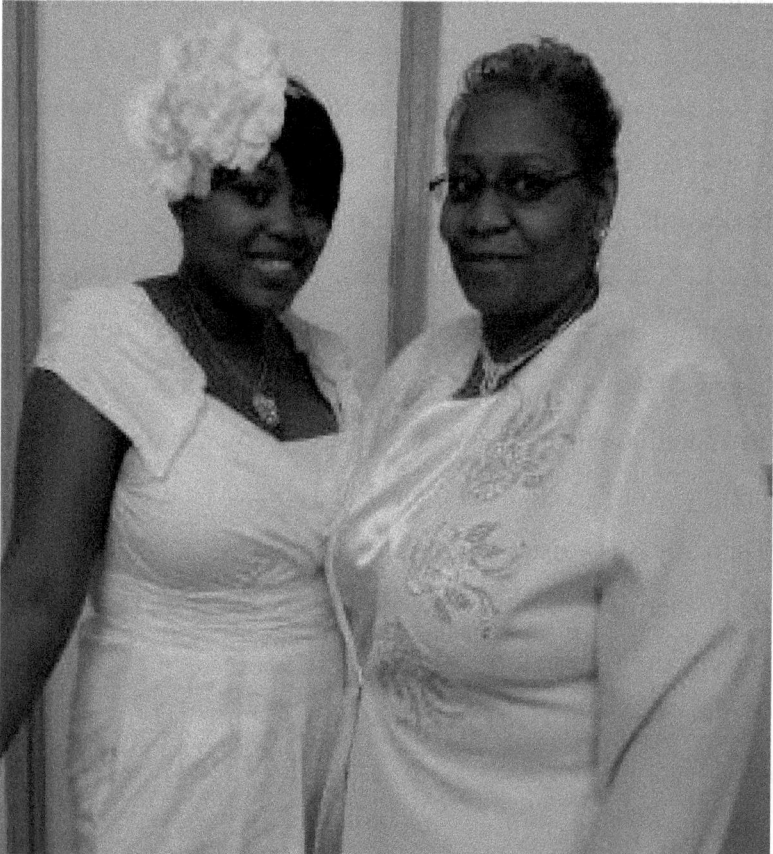

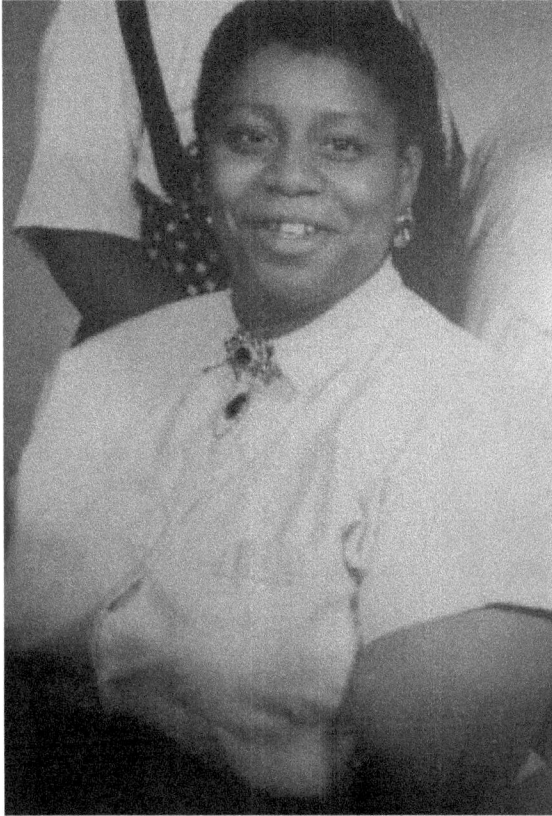

Sheila Byrd has been married for 30 years to Russell (Cordell) and has two children, Charles and Sheronne. She is an Entrepreneur and loves God with all her heart.

F.R.O.G.
(Fully Rely On God)

I have removed all of the negativity from my life.

If it's not positive and not for my benefit,

I don't want any parts of it.

Sarita Joy Jordan

F.R.O.G

(Fully Rely On God)

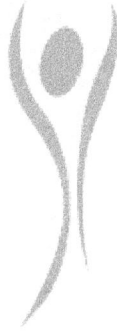

Two big, bulging eyes, long, apparently big feet, spotted, scaly, acne-prone skin and feeling "green." A single mother of one by the age of 21, but on my way to being the first college graduate in my entire family. After graduation in May 1990, my life was full of upsets and disappointments. I felt like I had no support from my family, was unemployed, recovering from a failed relationship and living day to day with low self-esteem. Nevertheless, those adversities became the "lily pads of my life", stepping stones. I began to hop from one lesson to another, always searching for happiness. For the next 15 years, I experienced many "lumps and

bumps." By this time in my life, I expected to have landed. However, when I didn't, I accepted the reality that it was another opportunity for GOD to show me His goodness. My feet were planted solidly when I realized that life's challenges were reminders to **Fully Rely On God,** *(F.R.O.G.).*

One fall day, in September 2005, a "lump" appeared that was unlike any trial I had ever faced. It was not painful. It was just there. It was the size of a small pea, big enough for me to see. I was later diagnosed with the big "C", Breast Cancer. "Ribbit!" I never questioned GOD, "Why?" Shortly thereafter, there were tests here and doctors there, like flies. I had to undergo surgery, chemotherapy and radiation with no hair, oh my!

Today, at the age of 43, I finally realize that I didn't have to kiss so many frogs trying to find my prince. All I had to do all along was fully rely on Him and I would be convinced. I survived the metamorphosis only to start life's process all over again! Yes, today is the first day of the rest of my life. I am living with a purpose and thriving!

I now have a rejuvenated approach to living beyond my 2005 Breast Cancer diagnosis: Stage One Invasive Ductal Carcinoma. I celebrate life in every which way I can. From travel, to just smelling fresh air, to exercise and diet. I know that if I make sure that my mind, body and soul are in sync, I could add some years onto my life. I spend a lot of my time volunteering at various non-profit agencies, telling my story to others to empower, educate and provide hope. I also spend quality time with my children; ages 23, 18, 12 and 5. As you read the ages of my children, you have probably noticed that I have a young child.

In December 2006, a year after my diagnosis, I discovered I was pregnant. I was in complete shock, because I didn't think I could get pregnant after Breast Cancer treatment. The Lord blessed me after Cancer, after surgeries, after chemotherapy, after radiation and after taking a drug, called Tamoxifen used to keep the cancer from returning. After chemo, I no longer got a monthly menstrual cycle. My Oncologist told me that if I didn't get my period within a year after treatment, I would go into early menopause and be unable to conceive.

My OB/GYN doctor feared the pregnancy could increase my risk for Cancer recurrence and advised me to terminate my pregnancy. Reluctantly, I signed the papers to have an abortion. This decision went against every moral that I believed in. I had to think about my own mortality. I questioned myself, "Do I go forward with this pregnancy, even though I already have three kids that depend on me?" "What if I don't make it through this process? How can I leave my children motherless?" After endless prayer and health considerations, I ultimately decided to keep the baby. I just couldn't go through with the procedure. I felt like my life had been spared for a reason, so who was I to make the decision to take another life?

At this point, I gave in and **Fully Relied On God**. Since my prenatal doctor didn't support my decision, I switched doctors. I visited with a team of specialists at the hospital where I received Breast Cancer treatment. After numerous tests and procedures to ensure the baby was healthy, my new doctor gave me a clean bill of health. The team concluded that there was no real medical reason, at that point, why I couldn't go forward with the pregnancy. I decided not to make a decision based on someone else's opinion, but to do what was best for me. In July of 2007, I gave birth to a healthy baby boy. My son, Jabaryi Mykai, which means brave, strong warrior in African Swahili, turned 5 years old on July 12, 2012. He is a blessing to me, as my story will continue to be a blessing to others.

About 3 years ago, I decided to take different steps to maintaining my health and have an active role in the management of this disease. I have altered my eating habits. I am eating more fruits and vegetables and have cut a lot of sugar from my diet. I used to drink bottles of Pepsi like water. I have replaced the soda with water and now Pepsi doesn't even taste good. Sodas now taste too sweet. While I thought I was ready to tackle exercise and diet, I enrolled in a Fit Study at a local University. After a comprehensive physical; I found that I was severely Anemic. Needless to say, I was NOT able to join the study. I returned to my Oncology team to discuss the Anemia and had to begin a lengthy process of receiving iron infusions intravenously. This entailed visiting the hospital 2 to 3 times a week off and on for 2 years. I began to think that I had to do something about my health. I didn't want to continue this regime for the rest of my life.

Last year, I joined the local gym in my neighborhood and even entered a weight loss contest. I had begun my journey. I lost about 15 lbs from changing my diet, walking, Zumba and other fit classes, just to name a few. My personal trainer even tried to get me to run, but that was a total failure. I hated running, so I thought. I couldn't breathe, I couldn't keep my balance on the treadmill, and it was a disaster. However, I still wanted to try it, but how? When?

As a regular user of facebook, I began to see some of my friends post on their status about their running experience. I would just read the messages and see posts and wish that I could do it, also. Running looked "freeing", just the remedy I needed to stay on task with my exercise goals. I had to do this because I want to be healthy. I have a burning desire to do anything that will grant me peace, tranquility and keep me away from the Oncology unit at the hospital.

"No more needles!"

"No more chemotherapy!"

"NO MORE! NO MORE!"

I have removed all of the negativity from my life. If it's not positive and not for my benefit, I don't want any parts of it. I want to remain stress-free, because stress and I don't get along. Therefore, it's not welcome in my world.

One day I inboxed a friend and told her that I want to run and asked, "How could I get started?" She said, "I run with a group called Black Girls Run (BGR)! Their mission is to encourage African-American women to make fitness and healthy living a priority. BGR's movement and I are a perfect fit, for more reasons than one. Not to mention I just love, love, love the PINK laces in my running shoes, for obvious reasons. My friend invited me to come. Still reluctant to go to a meet-up, I just continued to look at the pictures and the posts of the BGR group on facebook.

I was even watching the progress of a high school basketball mate, and was amazed at her transformation. I had no idea she had lost close to 100lbs. I noticed that she would always post her motto, "Movement is Medicine". I thought that was amazing. If my classmate had the courage to start moving, then what was my excuse? She looked so happy and was so dedicated to running, so I thought to myself. In June 2012, there was a posting asking for anyone who was interested in running to feel free to come to a new members meeting. This was the perfect opportunity, the change that I have been looking for. I showed up to the BGR meeting at Lloyd Hall in Fairmount Park. There were over 100 women that showed up interested in running.

After a 15 minute warm-up, I started off slow. I would walk some and jog some, which the group refers to as "wogging". I began to show up for meet-ups regularly. Within 30 days, give or take, I was able to run straight for 3 miles. That was such an exhilarating feeling! As a result, I am dedicated to continuing with running. I have benefitted greatly from this experience. Not only is the exercise trimming inches from my waist, the motivation and support from the women in the group is phenomenal. Their motto is, "No women left behind". I even ran in my first race this past July. I ran 4.5 hilly miles and completed the race in under an hour.

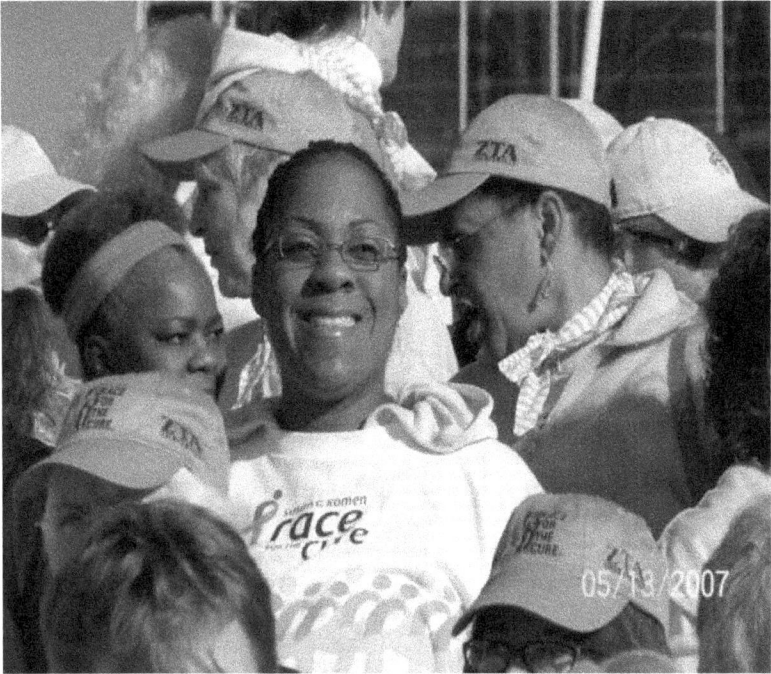

My purpose in life is to continue outreach and advocacy for other woman that may have to experience such an occurrence, like Breast Cancer. Now, I can add the health component to purposeful living as well. I will run in some of Breast Cancer awareness 5k races with the love and support of my BGR family. Lastly, but certainly not least, although I am losing weight, trimming my waist and thighs and feeling energized, don't get me wrong, I still have to see doctors regularly. Make sure you do to. However, I can do so, armed with knowing that I have chosen to take an active role in my ongoing recovery, while I strive to remain in remission. Currently, I am 7 years in remission and counting.

 In closing, although my life's road has been a difficult one, I am too blessed to be stressed. I have learned to enjoy the simple pleasures in life today, because tomorrow may never come. Try it, I think you would like it too. I am living proof. I am a living, walking, breathing, running testimony!

Remember, F.R.O.G.

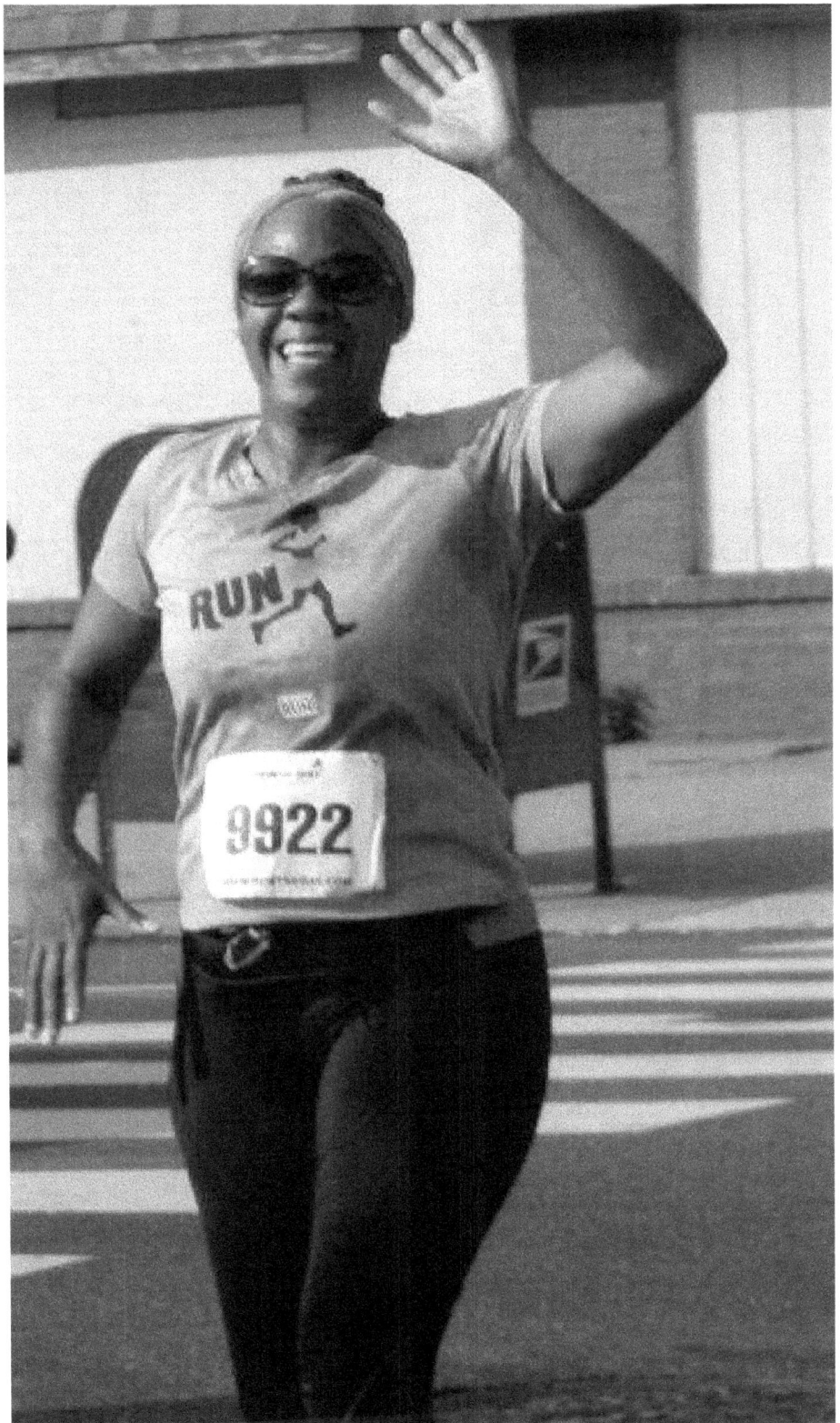

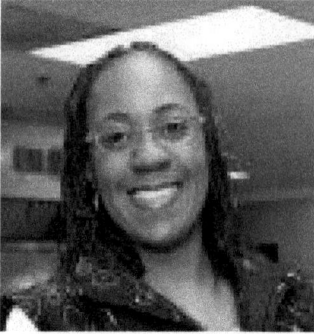

My name is *Sarita Joy Jordan*. I am a single mother of 4 children. I have two daughters and two sons, who range in age from 22 to 5 years old. I am a very active and involved parent because it's important to me that they have a strong foundation in which to be successful in life. As a result, my children will be very productive citizens, which they are currently being demonstrated in their own lives.

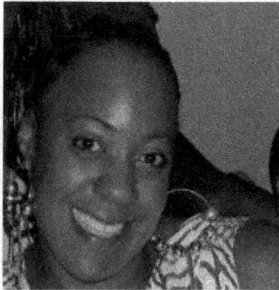

I graduated from college in 1990, with a Bachelor of Science in Management Information Systems. In May of 2005, I obtained a Paralegal Certification from Widener School of Law, Legal Education Institute program. For the past 10 years I have been employed in the Social Services field that included assisting clients with various needs to help them obtain the goal of self-sufficiency.

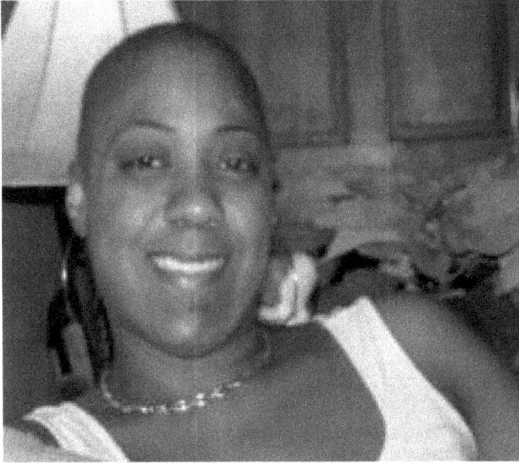

In 2005, I was diagnosed with breast cancer and was forced to retire from my job as a supervisor in the Department of Public Welfare. As I took the time to go through my treatment and healing process, I was able to figure out and fine tune what my life purpose should include. First and foremost, it would be to use my story as a testimony, to give others hope. Also, it would include volunteerism and advocacy for those that are unable to navigate the Health Care system themselves. I have always had the desire and passion to assist others. I am affiliated with various non-profit Breast Cancer support groups; i.e. Young Survival Coalition, Women of Faith and Hope, Praise Is The Cure, and Living Beyond Breast Cancer, just to name a few.

LIFE LONG JOURNEY

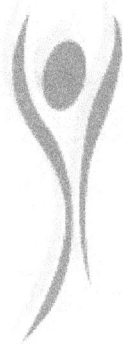

I have to accept that this battle
with weight won't be over
when I reach my goal.

It is a lifelong journey for me.

TINA GORDON-BROOKINS

LIFE LONG JOURNEY

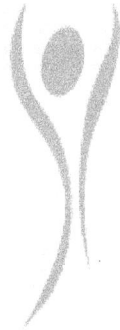

In my 47 years, I've learned a few things about losing, gaining and maintaining my weight. Yes, I am on the obese side on the weight charts. For people like me, who have what doctors say a "weight problem", the struggle goes on. At one point I lost 60 pounds and I felt very good, but I put it back on in a matter of five to seven years. At one point, I was heavier than I was after having my last child. It is a struggle just to maintain my weight, but I take it one day at a time.

MOVEMENT IS MEDICINE

My key scripture is Philippians 4:13

I can do all things through Christ who strengthens me

Knowing this, I know I can change my life style and eating habits. Currently, I log what I eat onto myfitnesspal.com. It is extremely beneficial for me. It calculates my calories, carbs, fat, protein, cholesterol, and sodium. It is just a reminder for me to keep control of my portions.

Over the past few years, I have experienced numerous ups and downs with my weight and I made up in my mind that I have to make life style changes. I wish I can say I have met my goal in weight loss, but I know it is one day at a time. I know I am doing all the correct things: tracking my food, walking (would love to run, but I was diagnosed with Rheumatoid Arthritis in 2011), not getting bombarded with stressful situations and seeking support from friends and family who are on my side.

I have to accept that this battle with weight won't be over when I reach my goal. It is a lifelong journey for me.

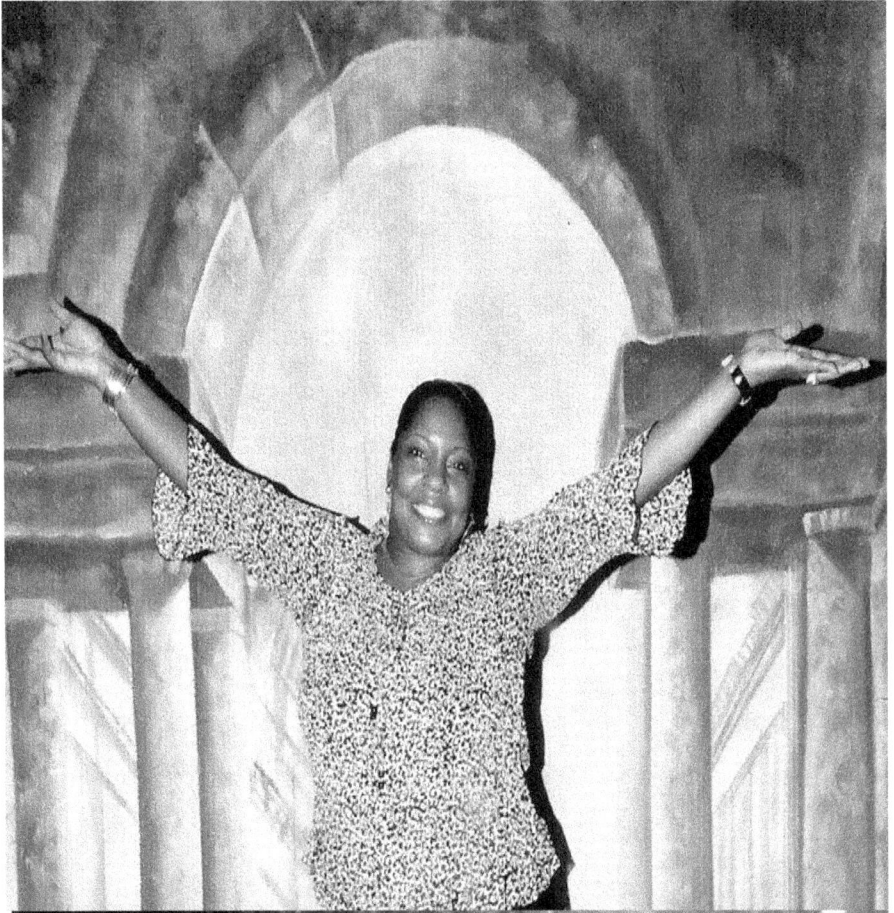

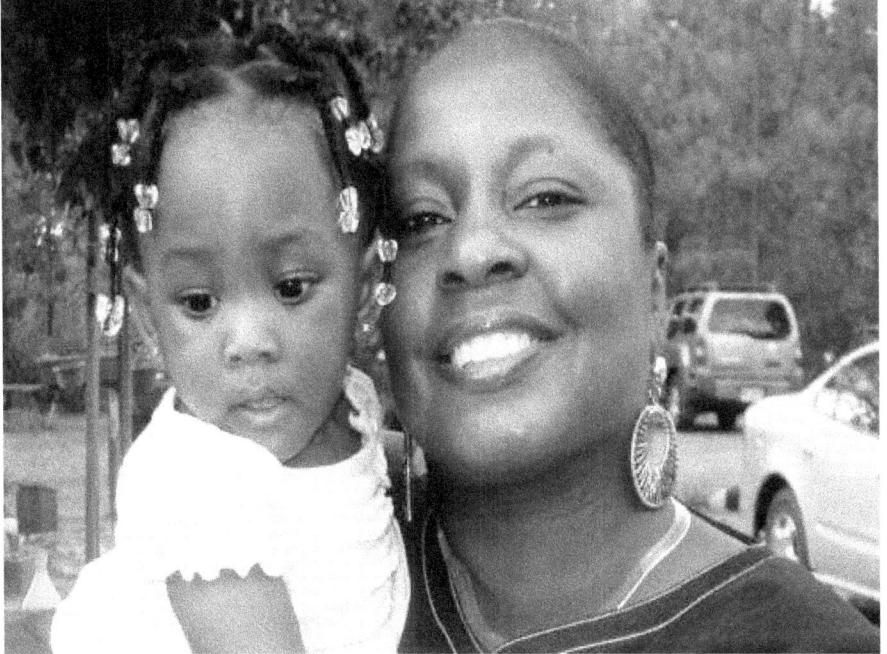

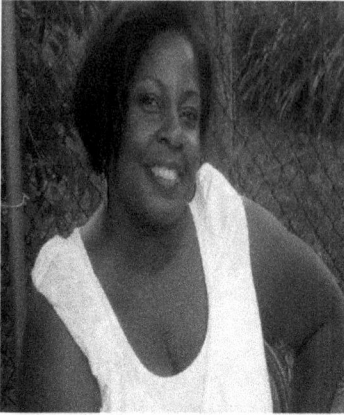

My name is *Tina Gordon Brookins*. I am a 47 year old mother of three children (Christian, Detrich, and Willis) and grandmother of six. I live in a small southern town called Sylvania, Georgia. I work as an assistant to a vice president for Academic Affairs at a major University.

I took care of my parent's for the past few years and my mother passed away on April 28, 2012. I now take care of my 89 year father, who himself stays quite busy. I attend Statesboro Mission Outreach Ministries, Inc., which I am heavily involved with and I work in its office. I volunteer with different organizations in my community, I love to travel, cook, and make special meals for my grandchildren (Jeremiah, Jasiah, Samuel, Solomon, Detrich, and Madison)

GET UP
AND *MOVE*
SOMETHING

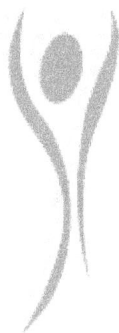

NOT A QUICK INSTANT FIX

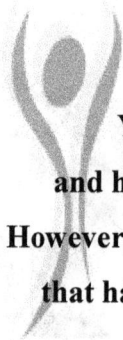

Weight loss surgery isn't a quick fix.
You will have good days and bad days
and have to work hard at the choices you make.
However, it is what you do with those days and the tool
that has been given to you that make a difference.

DENEEN YOUNG

NOT A QUICK
INSTANT FIX

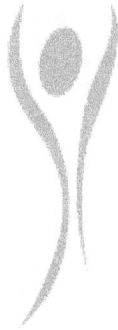

This has taken me forever to put on paper and share. I'm sure someone can relate to when you have pressed past some things in your life and then have to go back and relive or reflect on them. It can be major. Finally, I am not putting off "thank you" to myself and so many others who have been on this journey with me. As well as acknowledging those that have hurt me, knowingly and unknowingly (WOW, now that felt good). As I share some of my personal journey with you, my prayer is that it will bless someone to keep pressing and keep pushing. I also pray that it will educate you as well as push you towards becoming a better and healthier individual.

As I think back over my life, my journey leading up to becoming a runner as well as a better and healthier me, began about fifteen years ago. I began working on the "inner" me; mentally, emotionally and spiritually. Then the ultimate change came, the "tough love" conversation from my uncle. Next was identifying my 1st "tool", gastric vertical sleeve surgery. I discovered it didn't stop there. I implemented my next "tool", which was running. Then came the final stage, "push" and "press". This stage consisted of eating healthy on a regular basis, working out at least four days a week and being steadfast on changing my mind-set and lifestyle.

Snap shot of my story:

My journey began fifteen years ago. During the latter three years, I realized how much my weight was getting in the way of my life. I experienced panic attacks so intense, that I thought I was having a heart attack. I then began noticing my weight gain and my habit of eating out of fear, doubt, low self esteem and anxiety. Me? Low self esteem? I thought I had it all together. I was all that and a bag of chips. I knew I had a pretty face and could dress my behind off. However, deep down inside, I was holding in all the past hurts and pain.

SIDE NOTE: Whew! All the work, movement and the residue still takes you there for a second--okay breathe Deneen.

Now that the hurt and pain of the past had resurfaced, I began reliving being molested by four cousins from the age of seven/eight till about nine/ten years old. Two of them lived right here in Philadelphia and would actually come to visit our home often. The other two lived in Virginia. The molestations only occurred the summers my father would drop me off for a visit. That's another story for another time.

Another thing that resurfaced was my habit of searching for that "real love". I went from boyfriend to boyfriend but eventually realized they only wanted one thing. Unfortunately, that didn't become full circle until I started dealing with it all. I thought I was okay. I now had a husband that loved me and gave me all that I asked and wanted. I now had a baby boy (our miracle), a house and a car. I was set. But nope, all that didn't matter. I still had a void, low self esteem and wore a mask to hide it all. Finally, I was tired of the panic attacks and thought I was ready to get the pounds off. Little did I know, it wasn't the pounds that I needed lose, it was all the "weight" from the past that was holding me down and back from my future. It was me not loving all of me and honoring what God created. It was me not trusting God and living out my purpose that He had for me.

I finally went to a psychologist (male and a Christian) who helped me, in some ways, begin to figure things out. However, something was missing. I continued having panic attacks and repeating the same things over and over again, but in a different way. I wasn't allowing my husband to love me the way he needed and wanted. Everything was on my terms. I wasn't enjoying my life. I was still a perfectionist.

An example of that for instance: I would stay up on a Friday/Saturday evening and clean my house from top to bottom (like when you spring clean) until 3/4 am in the morning. I would get up on Sunday morning, go to church and not able to worship because I was so tired. However in my home; every pillow, every area of my hard wood floors was in place and in tip top shape for the human eye.

I began to open up and pray with my big sister, B. Michelle Horton. I listened to her wisdom and cried on her shoulder. I was introduced to a psychologist: This differed from my last experience in that she was a Christian and a woman. I stayed in therapy with her for well over four year, then on and off afterwards. I learned about how my anger and low self esteem issues I had kept me from not being able to love myself. The most important thing I learned to identify it and how to deal with it. I learned what God had to say about it all too. I learned that this experience was needed for my next journey.

One day, I was hospitalized with pneumonia and was told the morning after being admitted to the hospital, "You are one blessed woman. We expected you to be on a ventilator." I began to cry and promised myself I was going to get on track with my health and loose the weight. Well, that didn't happen. I tried again and again and again. Different tools and programs, but nothing worked. I finally gave up and accepted I would just remain overweight. I was miserable and began to make everyone around me miserable. I know I said I finally got it, but did I really?

My psychologist closed her practice and told me, "You are more than ready for the world. God is ready for you, so you don't need me any longer." OMG! I finally realized that we are all always a work in progress. This is where I started to know I had to keep pushing and keep pressing. Year before last, a co-worker shared she was having bariatric surgery. All I could hear was excitement in her voice. I shared my fears and she told me with such authority, "Deneen you will know when it is time for you to get on track. Find a tool and decide that you will do what you need to do for you to succeed. You have already begun by admitting what has been ailing you and have been working on you. That is the best thing".

I walked away thinking when and how will I know God? I don't understand why you have allowed so much pain to happen to me. I thought I could do this on my own, but maybe, just maybe God has a different plan.

Then it happened: in February of 2011 my uncle gave me a dose of "tough love". He asked, "Why are you killing yourself and what are you going to do about it? We all love you and want you here on this earth for a very long time! Don't you want to live long enough to see your grandchildren?" My response after pondering for a moment was, "I want to live long enough to see my great grandchildren!" This was like déjà vu! I had a dream, months, before about this very conversation! Everything he said to me over the telephone was what he said in the dream. I didn't tell anyone about the dream other than my husband. For me that was a move of God or the sign I was looking for.

Weeks after the "tough love' conversation, I went to my family doctor and shared my interest in bariatric surgery. She was thrilled and referred me to a surgeon, Dr. Tichansky at Jefferson Hospital in Philadelphia. My consultation was in

MOVEMENT IS MEDICINE

March of 2011. After long nights of prayer, I mean praying stretched out on the floor laying prostrate before Him, and conversations with my husband, children and my big sister/friend Michelle, I decided on the gastric vertical sleeve surgery.

For years I was like most I have experienced on my journey, uneducated about the whys, dos and don'ts. I took part in the very judgmental thinking: "oh they only want a quick fix" or only celebrities and white people do this. I educated myself and kept prayer in the forefront at all times with each step I took. It seemed like each step in my process was a breeze and I got clarity from Him.

Two of the most memorable steps for me occurred at the doctor's office and the support group meeting.

The receptionist had all of my paperwork ready for labs upon my leaving the consultation.

I said to her, "They told me to call back when I make a decision and then come back in for all of my paper work."

She says to me, "I have a feeling that it will all work out and you will need your paperwork now."

I'm looking at her face and share with her, "You seem so familiar to me. I'm glad you think I will be doing this. God will have to send me a sign and then I will know for sure".

We both start asking each other questions to figure out why she seemed so familiar to me. That day we weren't able to put our finger on it.

Fast forward—

I got my first sign immediately walking out of the office. I looked up and said, "Well Lord, if this is meant for me, then you will send me a sign because I know this "big behind" will not make it to get blood work done in time before they close in five minutes."

He answered me. I get to the lab and the hours had changed. They were open until 7 pm and it was now after 5 pm when they would have closed. The next time I visit the office, the woman behind the counter and I figured out why she was familiar to me. She was related to my cousin and I knew her since she was born, WOW look at God.

The other memory:

While attending my first support group meeting, everyone made me feel like I was part of the family. They shared their experiences with me, a lot like we do in my running group Black Girls Run. What sticks with me the most is my "team" (surgeon, nurse practitioner and my nutritionist) all shared: "If you do what we share with you to do, you will be successful. The key is, you must do the work and use the tool".

My "movement":

My surgery was on July 18, 201. Well to my surprise a month post surgery I had the urge and the motivation to begin to move physically, finally. I was eating the proper meals and portions, losing 20lbs. I realized I needed to add more to my healthy living plan. I began on my own to power walk/run 2-3 miles, line dance and Zumba almost every day without getting out of breath! I was able to walk up several flights of stairs and still breathe! For the first time in my life I actually looked forward to working out first thing in the morning! I've always been confident, but now my confidence level was up so high. I felt like "ME" again. That low self-esteem I was working on was through the roof! WOW! My constant prayer was, "Lord, keep me humble. I must continue to honor you in everything I do."

After one of my many morning posts on FaceBook after a walk, I was invited by a friend to Black Girls Run! Philadelphia. That was the best gift ever someone gave me. I immediately got on the BGR Facebook page, but guess what? I was talking only. I thought to myself, OMG these women are runners. I just want to get moving with someone so I can get these pounds off. I can't run. I can trot but not run with them. That's it, back to my track I go. Well, He had other plans for me. One evening, I remember a post on the page by our lead Ambassador, Jocelyn. She posted something about coming out even if you don't run and she would be there waiting. When I read that post my first thought was: that post is for me. Then I saw another post that the other Ambassador, Dawn, would be there too. Then yet another post from a member Marla. I'm thinking to myself, WTH? Okay, now you don't have any more excuses about being intimidated, it is up to you. You went through all of this to give up? No way, no how!

I finally made it out in the cold to my first meet-up with BGR in October! WOW, the Ambassador is walking and trotting with me. She is actually giving up her time to help me. Then the next time I'm out, I meet another member, Gina. WOW, a total stranger, so I thought, was talking to me. I discovered she knew my siblings, small world. We decided we would do this thing together. We were going to try out best to wog and set a goal to run. The next thing I know, I'm at meet-ups on a regular and Marla is right there waiting for me on the weekends to train and encourage me. Between her, Jocelyn and Dawn I could not believe what was happening.

NOT A QUICK INSTANT FIX

Okay side note: I am in tears as I am writing this reliving those moments thinking of ALL of the past pain and hurts. WOW God! Beauty for ashes, now I get it.

Then I meet Coach Leslie, that's what we call her, a gem. She starts sharing all of this information with me about my body and my work-outs. The ultimate thing that happened was that she helped me be okay with the fact that I used a tool that most African American women wouldn't, because of being uneducated and accepting being unhealthy. Her words moved me to the next level in my journey.

I took the steps to save my life and to be okay with my choice. She said, "Do you realize what you have done? You have saved and added years to your life. It doesn't matter what "tool" you have used. If we both use a different tool but both don't eat right and/or don't exercise. We both have the same results in the end, weight gain and an unhealthy lifestyle" WOW! I thought about that and realized she is right. I asked myself, "Why are you still walking around not sharing, not honoring God and being proud? You worked on the mental and emotional components. You know God gave you a gift with this "tool" that only He created and educated the doctors to use."

Next journey for me—

I honor and respect the choices that I made for me to save my life and to live longer. This journey has allowed me to be active with my children. I am now able to run around with them, play basketball, bowl, work out, just move and yes most of all run. I love every moment my feet hit the ground. I made the choice to make a positive change. I am 47 and I feel so much younger! Weight loss surgery isn't a quick fix. You will have good days and bad days and have to work hard at the choices that you make. It is what you do with those days and the tool that has been given to you that make a difference. This has truly been a positive journey for me and, unlike a year ago, I am not ashamed to say I had vertical sleeve surgery. It is because of that, I am now a runner!

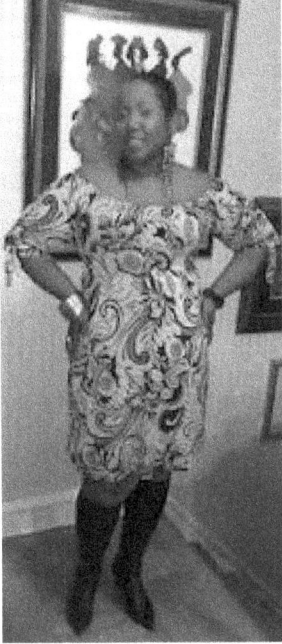

Sharing from your heart at times hurts, but the BLESSING is GREATER!

I will leave you with the closing that my Mary Kay consultants recite in a circle. When we say it out loud, in my mind I'm speaking to GOD saying, "Lord this IS MY LIFE as I am holding on to your unchanging hand."

I will let no one push my buttons

I will let no one rain on my parade

I will go over

I will go around

I will go through any obstacle that comes my way because I am highly motivated (FAVORED) truly dedicated and explosively successful!

MOVEMENT IS MEDICINE

So here I am, got some of it out and "whew", it wasn't bad. I like to greet the sun each morning with a run and a smile on my face. Like the song says "I'm Here", from the play *The Color Purple*--I love that scene and can relate to it. I am doing the darn thing. I am moving, I am pushing and pressing towards what my body can do, wants to do and what it craves do, to run! WOW, that sounds excellent! I am owning and honoring every part of my being. I am a runner. I am who I am supposed to be. This is the way I am suppose to be and the past is just that the past. I know there is always going to be a little residue to remind me where I came from, but to also let me know I can't and I won't go back.

Again, my story is not a "quick fix". My life is a work in progress and my journey keeps going towards staying fit and supporting this movement of "Movement is Medicine", BGR and the women in it. Whatever your goal is, if running is a part of it, know it can only take you as far as you allow it. You must honor each moment your foot hits the ground. You must feel each run and embrace all of you and without hesitation. You must live life to the fullest like it was your last day on earth. You must take care of your health because tomorrow my dear, is not promised. Now I would not be me if I did not leave you with this (yes in all caps) KEEP PRESSING and KEEP PUSHING! You are worth it! I know I am! Luv ya and let the journey continue!!!

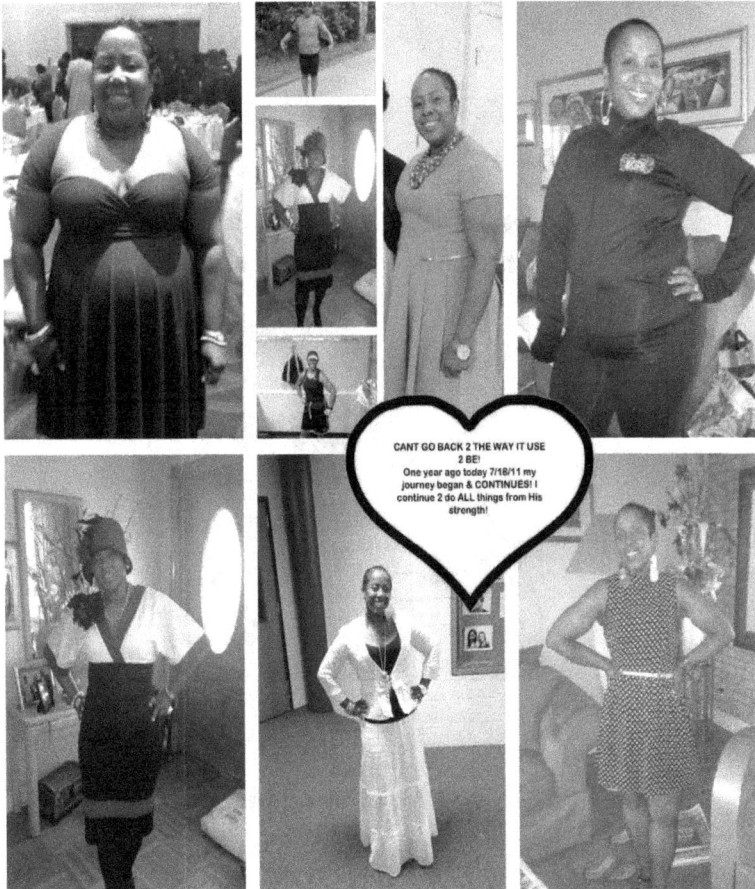

CANT GO BACK 2 THE WAY IT USE 2 BE!
One year ago today 7/16/11 my journey began & CONTINUES! I continue 2 do ALL things from His strength!

Before-Middle-After

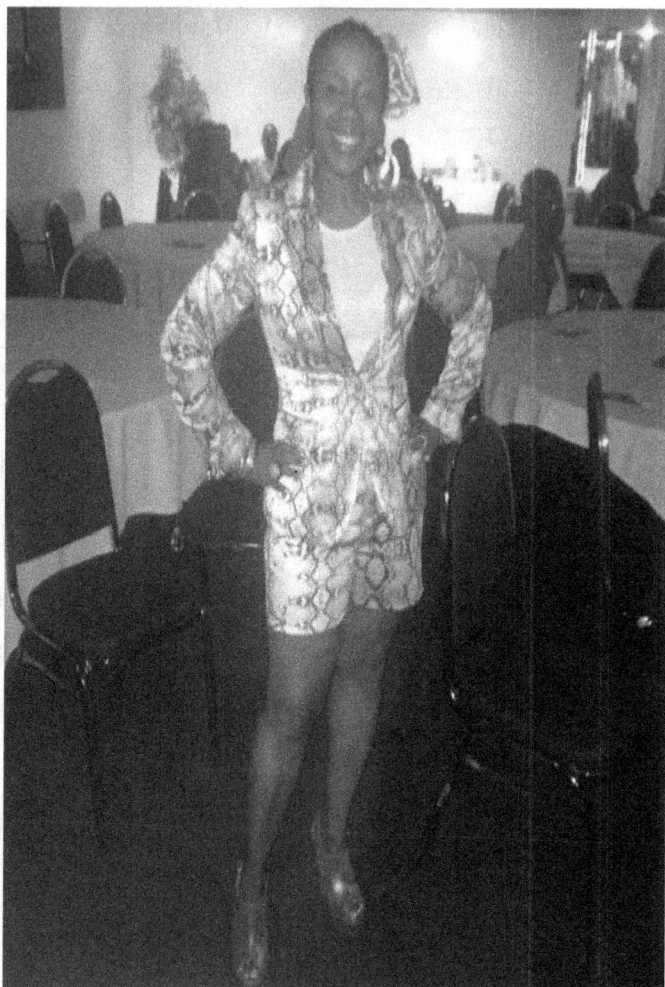

ME NOW: 119lbs gone!

http://thatgirlneen.blogspot.com/

Deneen R. Young is a wife and mother to two children ages 11 and 16. She loves the Lord and continues to strive for living a life honoring God. She currently works at an Independent Quaker School as well as owns her own business; *Neen's Closet Boutique*. She is the founder of Gurlz Get-2gether, an organization which provides an open forum and safe space for coaching, motivation, encouragement and support for girls ages 13 to 17 and women ages 18+ who have experienced low self-esteem and abuse and are willing to work on moving past the past.

Deneen's passion is running and Black Girls Run. Deneen began running in August of 2011 and joined Black Girls Run in November 2011. She became a Run Coordinator with BGR after two weeks of joining. In June of 2012, she became Co-Ambassador of BGR. Her other passion is helping people makeover themselves, mentally, spiritually, physically as well as with their fashion and style. Especially for people who don't have the time or interest to do it for themselves. A self-taught woman of God through life experiences, Deneen continues to push past the past and help others along the way.

Deneen was born and raised in Philadelphia, PA, She still resides there with her husband Michael and children KaMichael and Katelynn, who she counts it all joy to be her miracles. In her time off, she loves to travel to warm places with her family (which includes her mother and step-father) and run no matter what.

Deneen's belief and scripture she lives by is Proverbs 3:5-6.

"Trust in the Lord with all thy heart and lean not to thy own understanding. In all thy ways acknowledge Him and He will direct thy path."

For such a time as this!

GET UP AND *MOVE* SOMETHING

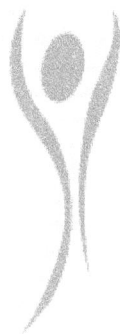

THAT GIRL NEEN's
BLOGS

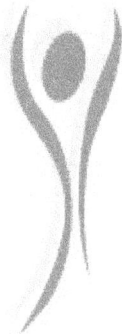

THAT GIRL NEEN'S

BLOGS

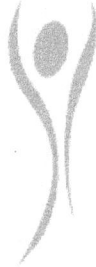

Here are a few shortened postings from my blog (www.thatgirlneen.blogspot.com/) that have been a blessing for me and prayerfully for you. It is not just about losing the weight of the pounds, but the weight that holds us bound. However, it is about running, wogging or walking--moving on so many levels (physically, mentally, emotionally and spiritually).

Journal Post:

Just a quick note this morning to share: I won't go back to the way it use to be. I have been healed. God's presence has changed me! What a great evening I had last night! You know I am thinking it feels good to CRY. I don't care what kind of cry you are crying or why you have those tears, but it feels good. I believe God smiles when we cry because He knows we are rejoicing in some kind of way. With that said, before I continue, what had me crying the other night as I came across a photo of myself, I believe was last year in November, I began to remember how stuffed I felt and even thought I was loving myself. I wasn't liking and loving me. Then I saw a recent photo of me and I'm like God! Thank you, just thank you for all that you have allowed! Here you go (before at 257lbs and mid-way about 51 pounds lighter more to go on the journey of pressing and pushing)! You just don't know! Not unless you have been on a journey and this journey. SMH! I am finding out so much about me and about others around me. Most importantly, getting closer to Him is a joy and the lessons along the WAY!

What was I thinking, thank God for BGR!

WTH was I thinking to sign-up for another race I know it was my new sister from another mother (my BGR sister Ily,

WOW). She sees more in me than I see in myself. "You got this Deneen Young," I said to myself. This morning was different from my other first races. I didn't feel like I was really prepared. Or was I prepared, and this is NOW WHO I AM?! I have accepted that THIS IS WHO DENEEN IS, a runner. Thanks to BGR, I am a runner, WOW!!!

Got to the Navy Base of the Gener8tion race and my BGR sisters are there already waiting. I am nervous and thinking, "How am I going to do 5 miles steady?" Okay Deneen, if you want to stop just start walking then pick it up again. Then I say to myself, "Well then you are cheating yourself and God because He keeps telling you He has you and you can do all things through Him!" So we are now all lining up at the start line and I'm with my sister Ily. I always look over at her and get that feeling like: WOW this sister here really loves me like a sister. She always gives me the THUMBS UP and says, "You ready? You got this!" Then I turn around and I see my other sister Mariel. She just gives me a smile that confirms that we got this. We START. WOW, I am remembering my student Emma saying, "Deneen remember walk and after the crowd thins out then start your run but at a slow pace." I FINALLY DID IT I DID IT! I AM HYPE I WALKED THEN STARTED RUNNING! The next thing I know, I'm with my girls. However, I can only see the back of them. In my ears I'm listening to the music. In my head I'm thinking to myself, "Nope, don't you dare. Keep your pace, slow moving, then you can pick it up on the turn around. So along the way I'm like man its getting hot then I see kids ages of my own children 11ish, 16, in between and older. I see women with strollers and I'm like, "Okay Deneen, do what God put in you." I get in the groove and I start running beside them encouraging them. Some LOL at me cuz I start singing my songs (no I can't sing). Some roll their eyes, but they get it going. They don't know it but me encouraging them out loud is me making me move and not think about the distance. Finally, I am at the turn around and thinking, "When is it going to be over? This is the longest 4.97 miles ever." Finally, I see the drill team again and then I see Mariel. I stick with her, just when my song comes on by Usher, "Bad Girl". I love that song! I start singing that out loud I mean real LOUD. This couple (teens) they are walking and I start dancing and running at the same time to get the girl to run. Finally, she does and she is LOL big time at me and then I get serious. After I leave them, I take off fast again. Okay Deneen, wait, you are out of breath, slow down. Nearing the finish line about a little over 1/4 miles, I see someone that looks familiar coming towards me. I look and it is Maxine (another BGR sister). OMG she finished and came back for me! The next thing I know Maxine is in my ear yelling, "Don't you stop Deneen! You have come too far! With God you can do all things through Christ that gives you strength!" I just shake my head. Then she tells me, "You better say that out loud!" I didn't want to and she yells even louder, "You can do what?!" I finally start repeating it real loud to the point I can feel my breath picking up. My legs are lifted higher and I am running so fast I can't believe it. OMG, I am running really fast. She then says, "Don't let that 57 minutes turn to 60!" Well, I looked at the clock and in seconds I was over the finish line! I couldn't stop running!

Well after all of that, I'm like God thank you for saving my life and allowing the vision of BGR to come just for me! Finally God, I got it. You continue to honor the desires of my life. I finally got my first official medal for a race what what... This black girl that runs is one hype sista!!!

This thing right here called BGR! Philly—is a movement a moment that continues with sisterhood, encouraging, supporting and lifting each other up!

Journal Post:

Things have taken place over the past few days and that's all I am going to say. I'm just sitting here telling myself as I will tell others, EMBRACE ALL that God has before you. Deneen, THIS THING RIGHT HERE CALLED LIFE/TESTIMONIES WOW! Sometimes I have those thoughts of going back or the bottom is going to fall out but I know I must embrace me where I am and know this is who I am and I am never going back. Yes, I am not perfect but continue to be a work in progress! I say all of this to share what is or has been in my head. I know someone else out there is thinking the same or has maybe fell off and went back. You can start over again and YOU HAVE CHOICES. We have to remain focused, embrace all of who we are and keep pressing. My students help me with that as I watch them and as I watch my own children deal with everyday life! For the first time, I'm looking at myself and thinking hmmmm, "I really, really like what I see and it is okay." We should do that. I'm feeling good about myself in so many ways and yes I am going to say it, RUNNING has helped take my self esteem to another higher level! I know I am a work in progress, but I say I must KEEP PRESSING and KEEP PUSHING TO EMBRACE ALL OF ME, PUSH AWAY WHAT AND WHO IS TRYING TO KEEP ME BOUND. I thought about a comment a few folks made, "You aren't still losing weight are you? You don't want to get too small. You don't want to be too skinny" WTH, what is too small? How about getting healthy to stay alive and live life to the fullest as my/our God wants me to do and as my family wants me to do as well!!! I work hard at eating right, exercise (running I so love) and have finally changed my mindset and my life style for good! So you my sista, keep pushing towards your journey of getting fit, living, loving and laughing out loud. We so need to keep enriching each other's lives. Stop saying you can't come out and move. Stop saying you can't walk or run. Do you know how blessed you are to have feet and legs that can move? I watched a man in a wheelchair and thought, wow that could be you or me. Do you know I pray over my legs and feet thanking God for them? Stop stuffing your feelings and your pain down your throat and do something about it, don't you want to live? Yup, I was there for years doing the same thing, stuffing all the past hurts and pain. However, now it's time I continue to pay it forward and help you to stop!!!! You must live! You have to live! Knowing and walking in the fact that you are fearfully and wonderfully made!! Wow, you gotta believe it and know it in your heart and with all of who you are!

GET UP
AND *MOVE*
SOMETHING

21 DAY
CHALLENGE

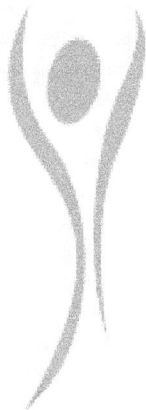

GET UP
AND *MOVE*
SOMETHING
DAY 1

Today's Date: _____ - _____ - _____

How do you *FEEL* today?

_____

_____

What did you *MOVE* today?

_____

What did you *EAT* today?

Breakfast _____

Morning Snack_____

Lunch_____

Afternoon Snack_____

Dinner_____

Dessert_____

How much *WATER* did you drink today? _____

Water intake (recommended daily: eight 8oz. glasses)

GET UP AND *MOVE* SOMETHING
DAY 2

Today's Date: _____ - _____ - _____

How do you *FEEL* today?

_____

_____

What did you *MOVE* today?

_____

What did you *EAT* today?

Breakfast _____

Morning Snack_____

Lunch_____

Afternoon Snack_____

Dinner_____

Dessert_____

How much *WATER* did you drink today? _____

Water intake (recommended daily: eight 8oz. glasses)

GET UP AND *MOVE* SOMETHING
DAY 3

Today's Date: _____ - _____ - _____

How do you *FEEL* today?

_____

_____

What did you *MOVE* today?

_____

What did you *EAT* today?

Breakfast _____

Morning Snack_____

Lunch_____

Afternoon Snack_____

Dinner_____

Dessert_____

How much *WATER* did you drink today? _____

Water intake (recommended daily: eight 8oz. glasses)

GET UP AND *MOVE* SOMETHING
DAY 4

Today's Date: _____-_____-_____

How do you *FEEL* today?

_____

_____

What did you *MOVE* today?

_____

What did you *EAT* today?

Breakfast _____

Morning Snack_____

Lunch_____

Afternoon Snack_____

Dinner_____

Dessert_____

How much *WATER* did you drink today? _____

Water intake (recommended daily: eight 8oz. glasses)

GET UP AND *MOVE* SOMETHING
DAY 5

Today's Date: ____ - ____ - ____

How do you *FEEL* today?

_____

_____

What did you *MOVE* today?

_____

What did you *EAT* today?

Breakfast _____

Morning Snack_____

Lunch_____

Afternoon Snack_____

Dinner_____

Dessert_____

How much *WATER* did you drink today? _____

Water intake (recommended daily: eight 8oz. glasses)

GET UP AND *MOVE* SOMETHING
DAY 6

Today's Date: _____-_____-_____

How do you *FEEL* today?

_____

_____

What did you *MOVE* today?

_____

What did you *EAT* today?

Breakfast _____

Morning Snack_____

Lunch_____

Afternoon Snack_____

Dinner_____

Dessert_____

How much *WATER* did you drink today? _____

Water intake (recommended daily: eight 8oz. glasses)

GET UP AND *MOVE* SOMETHING
DAY 7

Today's Date: _____-_____-_____

How do you *FEEL* today?

_____

_____

What did you *MOVE* today?

_____

What did you *EAT* today?

Breakfast _____

Morning Snack_____

Lunch_____

Afternoon Snack_____

Dinner_____

Dessert_____

How much *WATER* did you drink today? _____

Water intake (recommended daily: eight 8oz. glasses)

GET UP AND *MOVE* SOMETHING
DAY 8

Today's Date: _____-_____-_____

How do you *FEEL* today?

_____

_____

What did you *MOVE* today?

_____

What did you *EAT* today?

Breakfast _____

Morning Snack_____

Lunch_____

Afternoon Snack_____

Dinner_____

Dessert_____

How much *WATER* did you drink today? _____

Water intake (recommended daily: eight 8oz. glasses)

GET UP
AND *MOVE*
SOMETHING
DAY 9

Today's Date: _____ - _____ - _____

How do you *FEEL* today?

_____

_____

What did you *MOVE* today?

_____

What did you *EAT* today?

Breakfast _____

Morning Snack_____

Lunch_____

Afternoon Snack_____

Dinner_____

Dessert_____

How much *WATER* did you drink today? _____

Water intake (recommended daily: eight 8oz. glasses)

GET UP AND *MOVE* SOMETHING
DAY 10

Today's Date: _____-_____-_____

How do you *FEEL* today?

_____

_____

What did you *MOVE* today?

_____

What did you *EAT* today?

Breakfast _____

Morning Snack_____

Lunch_____

Afternoon Snack_____

Dinner_____

Dessert_____

How much *WATER* did you drink today? _____

Water intake (recommended daily: eight 8oz. glasses)

GET UP AND *MOVE* SOMETHING
DAY 11

Today's Date: _____ - _____ - _____

How do you *FEEL* today?

_____

_____

What did you *MOVE* today?

_____

What did you *EAT* today?

Breakfast _____

Morning Snack_____

Lunch_____

Afternoon Snack_____

Dinner_____

Dessert_____

How much *WATER* did you drink today? _____

Water intake (recommended daily: eight 8oz. glasses)

GET UP AND *MOVE* SOMETHING
DAY 12

Today's Date: _____-_____-_____

How do you *FEEL* today?

_____

_____

What did you *MOVE* today?

_____

What did you *EAT* today?

Breakfast _____

Morning Snack_____

Lunch_____

Afternoon Snack_____

Dinner_____

Dessert_____

How much *WATER* did you drink today? _____

Water intake (recommended daily: eight 8oz. glasses)

GET UP AND *MOVE* SOMETHING
DAY 13

Today's Date: _____ - _____ - _____

How do you *FEEL* today?

_____

_____

What did you *MOVE* today?

_____

What did you *EAT* today?

Breakfast _____

Morning Snack_____

Lunch_____

Afternoon Snack_____

Dinner_____

Dessert_____

How much *WATER* did you drink today? _____

Water intake (recommended daily: eight 8oz. glasses)

GET UP AND *MOVE* SOMETHING
DAY 14

Today's Date: _____ - _____ - _____

How do you *FEEL* today?

_____

_____

What did you *MOVE* today?

_____

What did you *EAT* today?

Breakfast _____

Morning Snack_____

Lunch_____

Afternoon Snack_____

Dinner_____

Dessert_____

How much *WATER* did you drink today? _____

Water intake (recommended daily: eight 8oz. glasses)

GET UP AND *MOVE* SOMETHING
DAY 15

Today's Date: _____ - _____ - _____

How do you *FEEL* today?

_____

_____

What did you *MOVE* today?

_____

What did you *EAT* today?

Breakfast _____

Morning Snack_____

Lunch_____

Afternoon Snack_____

Dinner_____

Dessert_____

How much *WATER* did you drink today? _____

Water intake (recommended daily: eight 8oz. glasses)

GET UP AND *MOVE* SOMETHING
DAY 16

Today's Date: _____ - _____ - _____

How do you *FEEL* today?

_____

_____

What did you *MOVE* today?

_____

What did you *EAT* today?

Breakfast _____

Morning Snack_____

Lunch_____

Afternoon Snack_____

Dinner_____

Dessert_____

How much *WATER* did you drink today? _____

Water intake (recommended daily: eight 8oz. glasses)

-235-

GET UP
AND *MOVE*
SOMETHING
DAY 17

Today's Date: _____ - _____ - _____

How do you *FEEL* today?

_____

_____

What did you *MOVE* today?

_____

What did you *EAT* today?

Breakfast _____

Morning Snack_____

Lunch_____

Afternoon Snack_____

Dinner_____

Dessert_____

How much *WATER* did you drink today? _____

Water intake (recommended daily: eight 8oz. glasses)

GET UP AND *MOVE* SOMETHING
DAY 18

Today's Date: _____-_____-_____

How do you *FEEL* today?

_____

_____

What did you *MOVE* today?

_____

What did you *EAT* today?

Breakfast _____

Morning Snack_____

Lunch_____

Afternoon Snack_____

Dinner_____

Dessert_____

How much *WATER* did you drink today? _____

Water intake (recommended daily: eight 8oz. glasses)

GET UP AND *MOVE* SOMETHING
DAY 19

Today's Date: _____ - _____ - _____

How do you *FEEL* today?

_____

_____

What did you *MOVE* today?

_____

What did you *EAT* today?

Breakfast _____

Morning Snack_____

Lunch_____

Afternoon Snack_____

Dinner_____

Dessert_____

How much *WATER* did you drink today? _____

Water intake (recommended daily: eight 8oz. glasses)

GET UP AND *MOVE* SOMETHING
DAY 20

Today's Date: _____ - _____ - _____

How do you *FEEL* today?

_____

_____

What did you *MOVE* today?

_____

What did you *EAT* today?

Breakfast _____

Morning Snack_____

Lunch_____

Afternoon Snack_____

Dinner_____

Dessert_____

How much *WATER* did you drink today? _____

Water intake (recommended daily: eight 8oz. glasses)

GET UP AND *MOVE* SOMETHING
DAY 21

Today's Date: _____ - _____ - _____

How do you *FEEL* today?

_____

_____

What did you *MOVE* today?

_____

What did you *EAT* today?

Breakfast _____

Morning Snack_____

Lunch_____

Afternoon Snack_____

Dinner_____

Dessert_____

How much *WATER* did you drink today? _____

Water intake (recommended daily: eight 8oz. glasses)

www.ingramcontent.com/pod-product-compliance
Lightning Source LLC
Chambersburg PA
CBHW072124270326
41931CB00010B/1660